"Brilliant in its simplicity and effectiveness, Dr. Wolf's book offers us truly healing and revolutionary medicine. Try it!"
—**Jack Kornfield, PhD,** author of *A Path with Heart*

"If you are living with any type of pain—be it physical or chronic, or stress in the mind or body—*Outsmart Your Pain* is a wonderful resource. Thoughtfully and compassionately written, this book will support and guide you in understanding your relationship to pain and the healing journey."
—**Sharon Salzberg,** author of *Lovingkindness* and *Real Change*

Outsmart Your Pain

Outsmart Your Pain

Mindfulness and Self-Compassion
to Help You Leave
Chronic Pain Behind

CHRISTIANE WOLF, MD, PhD

Foreword by Daniel J. Siegel, MD

THE EXP

NEW

The Experiment, LLC
220 East 23rd Street, Suite 600
New York, NY 10010-4658
theexperimentpublishing.com

This book contains the opinions and ideas of its author. It is intended to provide helpful and informative material on the subjects addressed in the book. It is sold with the understanding that the author and publisher are not engaged in rendering medical, health, or any other kind of personal professional services in the book. The author and publisher specifically disclaim all responsibility for any liability, loss, or risk—personal or otherwise—that is incurred as a consequence, directly or indirectly, of the use and application of any of the contents of this book.

THE EXPERIMENT and its colophon are registered trademarks of The Experiment, LLC. Many of the designations used by manufacturers and sellers to distinguish their products are claimed as trademarks. Where those designations appear in this book and The Experiment was aware of a trademark claim, the designations have been capitalized.

The Experiment's books are available at special discounts when purchased in bulk for premiums and sales promotions as well as for fund-raising or educational use. For details, contact us at info@theexperimentpublishing.com.

Library of Congress Cataloging-in-Publication Data

Names: Wolf, Christiane, author.
Title: Outsmart your pain : mindfulness and self-compassion to help you
  leave chronic pain behind / Christiane Wolf, MD, PhD ; foreword by
  Daniel J. Siegel.
Description: New York : The Experiment, [2021]
Identifiers: LCCN 2020057973 (print) | LCCN 2020057974 (ebook) | ISBN
  9781615197217 (hardcover) | ISBN 9781615197224 (ebook)
Subjects: LCSH: Chronic pain--Popular works. | Chronic pain--Psychological
  aspects. | Meditation--Therapeutic use. | Mindfulness-based cognitive
  therapy. | Awareness.
Classification: LCC RB127 .W65 2021 (print) | LCC RB127 (ebook) | DDC
  616/.0472--dc23
LC record available at https://lccn.loc.gov/2020057973
LC ebook record available at https://lccn.loc.gov/2020057974

ISBN 978-1-61519-721-7
Ebook ISBN 978-1-61519-722-4

Cover design by Beth Bugler
Text design by Jordan Wannemacher
Author photograph by Diana Feil Photography

Manufactured in China

First printing May 2021
10 9 8 7 6 5 4 3 2 1

*This is book is dedicated to every person
who lives with chronic pain.*

May you heal and be free from pain!

*And if that is not possible, may you find ease and
peace amid and despite everything.*

CONTENTS

Foreword by Daniel J. Siegel, MD xiii

Introduction: An opportunity to change your brain 1

PART 1: Caring for Yourself

1 You Are Not Your Pain 15
 MEDITATION: You are not your pain 20

2 The Pain Story 25
 PRACTICE: Writing reflection on the pain story 29
 MEDITATION: The pain story 31

3 The Box We Call Pain 35
 PRACTICE: Working with thoughts, sensations, and emotions 37
 MEDITATION: Opening the box of pain: exploring
 sensations, thoughts, and emotions 40

4 Self-Compassion for Pain 47
 MEDITATION: Self-compassion for pain 54

PART 2: Making Peace

5 Ending the War with Your Body   61
   MEDITATION: Kindness body scan   66

6 Finding Your Internal Support Group   73
   MEDITATION: Shared humanity: calling up
   the internal support group   78

7 Collecting Pearls   83
   PRACTICE: Collecting pearls   85
   MEDITATION: Yes, and . . .   88

PART 3: Handling Big Emotions

8 The Dark Clouds of Depression   95
   MEDITATION: Safe and pain free in the body   99

9 The Fear of Making Grief Real   103
   MEDITATION: Being with grief   107

10 Numbing Out   111
   MEDITATION: Urge surfing   116

11 Anger Is a Mixed Bag   121
   MEDITATION: Safely exploring anger   127

12 Freeing Yourself from the Prison of Resentment   131
   MEDITATION: Forgiveness   136

PART 4: The Pain of Connecting and Disconnecting

13 Dealing with Ignorance   143
   MEDITATION: Dealing with hurtful remarks   149

14 Loving Someone with Chronic Pain 153
MEDITATION: Equanimity: every person is on their
own life's journey 159

15 Finding Your People 165
MEDITATION: Finding strength and joy in connections
with others 169

PART 5: Shifting Perspective

16 The Comparing Mind 175
MEDITATION: Releasing your comparing mind 178

17 Making Meaning 183
MEDITATION: Making meaning: silver lining
backward and forward 188

18 The Paradox of Doing Nothing 193
MEDITATION: Doing nothing 197

19 The Big Picture 203
MEDITATION: The big picture 206

20 Stop Trying to Get Better 211
MEDITATION: OK as you are 215

Epilogue: Closing Thoughts 218

Resources 220

Acknowledgments 222

About the Author 224

FOREWORD

DANIEL J. SIEGEL, MD

IN YOUR HANDS is a powerful, clear, and practical guide to shifting your way of living with the experience of pain within your own body—or in the lives of those for whom you are providing care and healing. With extensive experience as a physician and meditation teacher, your capable and compassionate guide, Dr. Christiane Wolf, offers the gift of simple summaries of the science and practical aspects of pain and how our mind handles these experiences. The meditations—mental exercises— found here can transform how you live with pain.

You may be wondering: If pain is present in our bodies, how might a meditation help us develop a way of living with it?

Pain is mediated in a region of the human brain called the dorsal anterior cingulate cortex, whether somatic (in the body) or social (in our relationships). When pain is processed it creates an internal sense of hurt that carries the message: This is important, uncomfortable, and should be corrected. But if this pain, whatever its origin, is "in the brain," how can something we do with our mind—such as a meditation, an attitude, or an intention—shape how we experience that pain?

Meditation can be simply understood as an exercise that trains the mind. And the mind has many important pieces: how we experience sensations and emotions, called "first person," or "subjective," experience; how aware we are of that felt sense of life; how we process information, make meaning of our experiences, understand life, and share that with others; and how we regulate our emotions, thoughts, intentions, and narratives.

In this magnificent guide, you will find time-tested ways to support your own mind and face pain with more resilience, clarity, and purpose. Studies of how the brain registers pain after meditation training have shown that not only will the intensity of pain you feel diminish, but the ways your brain mediates pain will also decrease.

This valuable book will give you steps to change your relationship to pain for the better. The sensation of pain, when coupled with the resistance of the mind to accepting it fully as part of your life, leads to a magnification of your distress, which we can simply call "suffering." Mental suffering is amplified by our resistance to accepting things for what they are. At the heart of the powerful practices you're about to learn is compassionate acceptance. This mental state of receptivity is far from the passive "there's nothing I can do" state that some initially imagine when they consider this notion of acceptance. Ironically, acceptance is really about opening to things as they are right now. In the course of such receptivity, the resistance subsides, the suffering is radically reduced, and the pain creates less havoc in a person's life.

When pain is in our lives, naturally we would like it to go away. But commonly, and sadly, we resist approaching that sensation with full acceptance, which intensifies our suffering, and in turn makes our minds even more distressed and less able to think clearly, absorb other aspects of life, or find gratitude for just being alive. When our attention is narrowed around pain, the broader view of *placing pain in perspective* is lost. We can become consumed by the pain itself and may even "identify" with the pain as the totality of who we are.

These truths and practices will shift your perspective and your way of relating to pain in life. You are about to be invited to make mind training your own with a program that research suggests will enhance the quality of your life in meaningful and lasting ways. Enjoy!

INTRODUCTION

An Opportunity to Change Your Brain

WE ARE IN THE MIDDLE of an unprecedented pain epidemic and a related opioid epidemic. There have never before been so many people struggling with chronic pain or higher demand for pain relief. Today, the leading form of pain relief is pharmacological—and while the existence of pain medication is without a doubt a blessing, its use also comes with many unwanted side effects, including potential addiction to opioids.

The Centers for Disease Control and Prevention (CDC) state in their 2016 recommendations that "non-pharmacologic therapy and non-opioid pharmacologic therapy are preferred for chronic pain." Alternative treatments such as mindfulness and compassion practices, then, are paramount to fighting the epidemic, but they are not yet widely accessible as a treatment for chronic pain.

Over the past several decades, mindfulness and compassion practices have entered the mainstream and are now introduced and prevalent in settings as diverse as schools, workplaces, community centers, and government offices. They're being adapted for use by doctors and nurses, athletes, police officers, firefighters, and in the military, as well as for veterans with post-traumatic stress disorder. One of the biggest arenas for the application of mindfulness is in health care, especially but not exclusively in mental health treatment. Mindfulness-based interventions are increasingly accepted as evidence-based practices, supported by a growing number of health-care insurers and health-care professionals. Each year there are more scientific studies of mindfulness than the year before: While there were a handful of articles published in scientific journals on mindfulness in 2000, by 2018 there were nearly 850.

Mindfulness practices are increasingly popular because they are effective, easy to learn, and have few, if any, side effects. The most common so-called side effect is that "it gets worse before it gets better." Why is that? Because as we turn toward our experience, instead of turning away, we start to understand and feel what's been there all along. This practice teaches us the equation:

$$suffering = pain \times resistance$$

In other words, if we resist an experience like pain, or worry about it, our overall struggling and suffering increase. And while we often can't change the pain, we can change the level of resistance.

If this realization feels too overwhelming, simply back off. Go slower. Take baby steps. It's OK to be a slow learner!

I encountered mindfulness and meditation as a young adult while looking for a spiritual path and a deeper meaning to life. Many people helped me find my way, including some Buddhists who also practiced Insight Meditation. I was taken in by the relaxed, loving, and joyful way they showed up in life, and I started practicing and studying these ancient wisdom teachings. Entering medical school and then doing my residency as a gynecologist at the university hospital in Berlin, Germany, these practices helped me stay sane and grounded through many, many hours of rigorous training. I specialized in gynecological oncology, where dealing with emotional and physical pain is a daily occurrence. My meditation practice helped me become a better physician by allowing me to be more fully present with patients and their families—to listen deeply to the fullness of their experience no matter where the course of the cancer was taking them.

Back then I never taught meditation to my patients because secular mindfulness wasn't as well known and accepted as it is today. I wished, though, that every patient and everyone around them affected by the cancer could have these amazing tools to learn how to hold all of life in loving awareness.

In 2003, my husband and I, with our then five-month-old daughter, moved to Los Angeles "for just one year." Now, seventeen years later, we are still living in Los Angeles and—to my own biggest surprise—I never went back into gynecology. While the process of moving on from that career was long and did not unfold easily, but which I loved dearly nevertheless, I found a new central focus for my professional life. I became an Insight Meditation teacher and discovered the power of secular mindfulness, becoming a teacher and teacher-trainer for Mindfulness-Based

Stress Reduction (MBSR), the transformational program Jon Kabat-Zinn, PhD, founded in 1979 that has since spread worldwide. Since 2005, I have been teaching mindfulness classes for people who suffer from chronic disease and pain, and have been learning and growing together with my students ever since.

Because English is not my first language, I am acutely aware of the power, importance, and pitfalls of translation. My goal, then, is to translate complex practices and theories of these ancient wisdom traditions as well as scientific concepts into clear and easy-to-understand language—and to make the practices relevant and applicable to you, the reader of this book.

How can mindfulness and compassion help you with chronic pain?
Pain is a complex experience in which the *physical* component plays a major role, but not the only one. The two other main players are as follows:

1. emotions, how we feel about the pain, such as anxious or resentful, and

2. thoughts about the pain, which we call "the pain story" (what happened, what went wrong, what that means for our future, and so on).

The three components influence each other significantly: If we are able to lessen the impact of emotions and the pain story, we can lessen the overall level of pain experienced. This is how mindfulness can help.

Compassion eases pain by bringing a loving or caring presence to the painful experience. We all know how good and healing it is to feel compassion from another person, whether a loved one, a nurse, or a doctor. Many people find it hard to be compassionate to themselves, but it can be just as therapeutic as from another person, so it's a worthwhile skill to learn. Together, mindfulness and compassion are powerful allies to have on your healing team.

Many patients wonder: Will mindfulness free you of your pain for good? I honestly can't say, since each person's journey is unique. I have seen some patients' migraines, back pain, and other pains resolve completely with this approach after a just a few months, almost miraculously. Most people who engage in these practices in a serious and committed way find relief, calm, renewed energy, and joy. I have also seen virtually no change in some others. Pain is too complex for an easy fix, however much we wish for it. There is strong evidence that trauma, especially repeated childhood trauma, is connected to an increase in physical symptoms and disease in adulthood. How could it not be?

We know about the devastating effect of chronic, toxic stress on the body. The practice of mindfulness and compassion is a doorway into unwinding and releasing stress. When stress levels decrease, it can be felt in all three of the major players: thoughts, emotions, and physical sensations. The practices you will learn in this book are meant to be complementary to other methods that you have found helpful on your healing journey.

Is the goal of mindfulness to get off all pain medication?
This is such a common question! No, getting off all pain medication is not the goal. I have often seen people who think that this is the goal get stressed-out in their meditations. This belief also suggests that as long as you are on medication, you are a bad/not-good-enough meditator. In my

experience, meditation and medication work really well together. It is true that mindfulness practitioners often find that they can lower their dose through regular meditation and get more of a "feel" for how much is enough and when more is needed. As the emotional pain decreases through the practices mentioned here, so does the dosage of their meds. Often, people can go off of their medication for longer periods of time or can switch to an as-needed basis. This is true not only for pain medication but also for those that treat insomnia and for mood-stabilizing drugs.

HOW TO USE THIS BOOK

You can read this book chapter by chapter or in any order and try the suggested practices as you feel drawn to them. The chapters are intentionally short in order to give an overview of which practices people I've worked with have found the most helpful to offer relief of their pain symptoms.

In each chapter you will find a mindfulness or compassion concept and a personal experience of someone suffering from chronic pain. Each story is a conglomerate of several real people I have worked with over the years, combined here in order to protect their privacy. I learn best from this combination of theory and personal example. Each chapter closes with a guided meditation or practice. You can either read through the entire book first and then go back to individual chapters or take your time and explore one chapter and practice at a time. After a few chapters, the meditations will feel familiar. The meditations can be read but

I've found that for most people listening to an audio recording of them works best. An audio recording of each of the twenty guided meditations in this book is available for you to download. To access the audio files, visit christianewolf.com/oyp/audio, or scan the QR code below with the camera on your phone or a QR reader app:

Some chapters suggest that you see the experience of pain in a different light. Such practices give some people an instant aha moment and a shift in perspective. Others you may need to reflect on, discuss, and challenge over time. As they say, "Rome wasn't built in a day," and it can take time to change a lifelong belief about "how life works" or "who I am" as a person. One of the most encouraging discoveries of neuroscience is that we can indeed change our internal wiring and our views by exercising new ways of seeing and thinking.

THE MEDITATIONS

The basic setup of each meditation is the same
Set aside some uninterrupted time during which you do nothing but meditate. The meditations in this book each take 10 to 15 minutes. You can read the meditations slowly to yourself, pausing between each sen-

tence, but it's recommended that you listen to the audio recordings. If you'd like, you can even record them yourself and listen to your own voice! This can be especially powerful with the self-compassion practices.

Posture

Find a posture that invites ease and comfort, but not sleepiness. This can be sitting or lying down. You can also do a meditation standing up. Dining room chairs are usually better than a sofa as their seat is higher and they support a straight back. Make sure your feet are firmly planted on the ground. If your feet don't touch the ground naturally, put a blanket under them. Your hips should be at the same level as your knees, or even higher than the knees. Putting an extra cushion on the seat of the chair will do the trick to lift your hips. Try positioning your body in different ways.

While you might want to just sit with a straight back, without any back support, try placing a rolled-up blanket or yoga mat at the small of your back and then push back to lean against the back of the chair. This helps the spine to rest in its natural curvature.

If sitting is not a good option for your body, then you may lie down—or be in any position that alleviates the pain, really. You might want to give the "astronaut's pose" a try, where you rest your lower legs at a right angle on the seat of a chair while you lie down on the floor in front of it.

You can rest your hands anywhere you like.

Experiment with your eyes closed or with a lowered gaze. What helps you to stay more present?

Meditation 101

Start by feeling the feet on the ground or whatever they are touching. Then feel where the rest of the body is in contact with the chair, the bed, or the floor. Let yourself be held by those surfaces.

Then find where you feel your breath in the body. Where is it the strongest? At the nose, the chest, the belly? Use that as your anchor, the place you keep coming back to over and over whenever your attention has moved somewhere else.

Take a few longer, deeper breaths as you start your meditation. Then let the breath flow naturally.

Expect your mind to wander off topic. That's the nature of the mind. When you notice your attention is somewhere else, simply bring it back without judging yourself.

THE PRACTICES

The practices are like guided reflections on a particular topic. It is helpful to also set aside a bit of time for them. You might find it helpful to start with a short, 5-minute meditation on the breath so that the mind settles a little, and then do the practice. It's also helpful to journal after the reflection to track your experience with the practice.

My hope for you is that this book inspires you to use these time-tested methods to change your brain—and your pain—for the better!

In the midst of winter, I found there was, within me, an invincible summer.

—ALBERT CAMUS

PART 1

Caring for Yourself

1

You Are Not Your Pain

AS HUMAN BEINGS we tend to identify with whatever is significant in our life. We identify with our profession: "I am a carpenter . . . a lawyer . . . an entrepreneur . . . an artist" or with our marital or family status: "I am a wife . . . a father . . . an older sister . . . an only child." Such affinity is natural and usually not a problem. It helps us move through the world, supplies a perspective that helps us make decisions, and gives us a sense of belonging.

We also do this with recurring emotional states; for example, "I'm a happy person," "I'm a worrier," or "I'm an anxious person," and with physical states, like chronic pain. If you suffer from chronic pain, there is a good chance that at some point you will start thinking to yourself, "I *am* my pain" or "I *am* a pain patient." The mind moves from "In this moment I am experiencing pain" to "I *am* the pain."

One of the most helpful mental shifts that can happen for a pain patient when they start practicing mindfulness is realizing that you are not your pain. Your pain is *part* of your experience, but it is not defining or reducing you. When a pain sufferer gets that message, they realize they are so much more than their pain! They learn to take a step back and observe the pain instead of identifying with it—and to experience pain one moment at a time instead of becoming the pain.

Allie came to me with serious back pain. An accountant for a local law firm and the mother of a teenage boy, Allie had to stop working after her second back surgery didn't bring the hoped-for results. When she was in any position for longer than a few minutes, the pain intensified, so she couldn't work at her job anymore and was put on disability. Pain medication brought some relief, but Allie was afraid of becoming addicted to opioids, and she also didn't like the "checked-out feeling" that was a trade-off for getting the pain under control. Allie felt hopeless and anxious about her future. She said, "I'm a different person than I used to be. It feels like I'm broken now. It feels like the pain is a kind of monster that has become me."

When someone reaches this point, their perception changes from experiencing pain in this moment to a permanent state of being the pain or the person with pain. For some, it starts to feel like the pain has become a part of you, like your eye color or your ears—or even your whole body! When you *are* the pain, there are different and much more serious implications than if you are simply *experiencing* the pain.

Since we can't change what we are, we're stuck with the pain in the same way that we're "stuck" with the color of our eyes. The pain has taken up permanent residence in our being and become an inseparable part of who we are. Or so it feels. We'll start to think, talk, and behave as "the pain patient," and even say things like "people with [my sort of] pain don't do [insert activity]." This quickly turns into a habitual pattern of relating to ourselves—and the world around us—through the pain-patient lens. And it can lead to our ignoring what is true and what is right in *this* moment.

Identifying with the pain immediately makes our world more restricted. This has big implications. It might make us feel that there is something fundamentally wrong with us, or that we are defective or broken. We might even stop liking ourselves or lose trust that we are lovable the way we are!

Allie confirmed that she felt like she had turned into "this broken pain person." To help her, I asked her to start noticing when she was internally talking about her pain, to let go of that inner commentary for an instant, and to just "feel into" the actual pain of that particular moment as best she could. And continue to explore that feeling. I helped her find a sentiment that resonates with her, something to say silently to herself like, "This is a moment of pain," or simply, "Back pain. This is what back pain feels like." And to take a deep breath.

How you talk to yourself matters. As the saying goes, "Pay attention to how you talk to yourself because you are listening!" Instead of saying, "I'm in pain" or "I hate my back pain!" use more impersonal phrases like "This is a moment of pain." You're shifting to a different perspective, one that makes it "not about you." See how this makes a difference.

When I asked Allie to talk about the effect of using new language she said, "It feels lighter, not so close-up, not so personal. There is a sense of relief."

Being able to take our experience less personally is a key element in mindfulness practice. Whatever happens is always simultaneously personal and not personal. If this sounds paradoxical to you, you're right. That's because it's always about the perspective from which we are looking.

An often-told story from India illustrates this point beautifully. There once were four blind men who had never before encountered an elephant. One day an elephant was brought to their small town and they got to meet it. They were all led to the elephant at the same time and each felt a different part. The first one, grasping its trunk, said, "An elephant is like a thick, flexible hose." The second one, taking hold of its ear, said, "No, an elephant is a like a big leaf or a fan." The third one wrapped both arms around the elephant's leg and said, "No, an elephant is like a huge column or a tree trunk." And the fourth one, patting its side, said, "No, it's like a huge wall." We smile at these narrow views, each man experiencing the elephant in a limited way, but aren't we doing the same with our experience all the time?

Let's say you experience neck pain. Of course, it's your neck that has the pain. You know your pain's history and its impact on your life. But at the same time, it's just neck pain. Millions of people suffer from neck pain. Millions of people have the same or a very similar history and impact on their life. While most people hate their neck pain, it is not a mistake. There is nothing wrong with *you* that you suffer from this pain. Some human bodies develop neck pain, others don't. That isn't to imply that your pain doesn't matter. It matters a lot! I am inviting you to notice the impact of taking your pain *only* personally—as "my pain"—and I am inviting you to notice what happens when you broaden your perspective to "the pain in this moment."

After a few mindfulness sessions with Allie, I led her through another exploration. I started by asking, "Is that part of you that is aware of the pain also in pain?"

Allie looked at me puzzled. "What do you mean?"

"Didn't you tell me that you are aware of the pain?"

"Yes," she replied.

"So, can you go inside and check if the awareness of the pain is *also in pain*?"

Allie was curious and closed her eyes to pay closer attention to her experience. After a short while she opened her eyes again and looked surprised. "No," she said slowly. "That part of me that is aware of the pain is not in pain. That's so interesting!"

In meditating, I guided Allie to focus in on the observing aspect—the part that's aware of what's going on—and to let that become bigger in her experience. It's like shifting the load of attention from *being* in pain to *the awareness* of being in pain.

Over the next few months Allie continued to work on the way she talks to herself about the pain as well as shifting her perspective of it, which slowly changed both her relationship with it and the pain level itself for the better. "I am not the broken pain person anymore," she told me. "I am a person who experiences pain on a regular basis. And while it limits some things I can do, it doesn't define me at all. I feel a lot more at peace with the pain and at ease in my life."

You are not your pain

Find a comfortable position.

Maybe make some small adjustments to allow the body to be as relaxed as possible right now.

Pause.

If you are in a seated position, feel your feet on the floor—simply feel the ground under your feet.

If you are lying down, feel any pressure of the bed, sofa, or floor against your heels.

Feel where your legs are in contact with the chair or the bed. Notice where there is touch and where there is none.

Do the same with your back—notice if your back is touching something, like the back of the chair.

Now feel into what your hands are touching: maybe your legs, maybe one hand is touching the other.

Pause.

Move the attention to where you can feel the breath in the body.

Is it mostly at the chest or the belly? Can you feel a sense of expansion and contraction?

Follow the rhythm of the breath. When you notice your attention moving somewhere else, gently bring it back to feeling the breath in this moment.

Now notice if and where there are unpleasant or painful sensations in the body. Notice if it's one area or several.

Pause.

Choose one area to work with today.

Check in with yourself if it feels OK to start paying kind attention to the pain in this moment. If it feels too much or too overwhelming, just stay with focusing on the sensations of the breath and let the pain be in the background.

If you choose to work with the pain today, please bring a gentle sense of presence to it. Allow yourself to move a little closer or to step back as needed so that it feels doable and not forced.

Pause.

Notice if you start to tense up, as if to brace yourself for the impact of the pain. See if you can relax the muscle tension some. Explore also using the breath, letting go of tension on the exhale.

It can be helpful to imagine guiding the breath into the area of pain or around it, as if you are holding it in awareness, surrounding it with awareness.

The breath can be like a handrail for the attention.

Be gentle with yourself. Feel into the appropriate amount of attention.

Keep breathing.

Keep softening.

Pause.

Notice if there is an inner commentary like "I'm in pain" or "I hate this pain!" If there is, let that go for a moment and see what happens if you name what you are experiencing. Try it in a friendly, nonjudgmental tone, like "This is a moment of pain." "This is what (whatever pain you are feeling right now) feels like."

Pause.

It is not *my* pain, just *the* pain. Human beings experience pain. Many people experience exactly this kind of pain in this moment.

Pause.

Allow yourself the time you need to feel into this exploration of pain.

Keep breathing.

You can either just stay here or, if you like, move to another exploration.

Pause.

Now ask yourself: "Is that which is aware of the pain also in pain?" You can do this if you are feeling into the pain directly or if you are staying aware of pain in the background.

"Is the awareness of the pain in pain?"

Drop this question into your mind, as if you were dropping a pebble into a well, just feeling into the widening ripples instead of trying to think of an answer.

Pause.

When you are ready, let go of any questions and any explorations and come back to feeling the whole body, lying or sitting here.

Just the breath, the body, and awareness.

Pause.

In a few moments our meditation will come to an end. Take your time to transition, to open your eyes if you have them closed, and maybe stretch the body any way it likes right now.

2

The Pain Story

PETER WOKE UP to his alarm. As he opened his eyes, there was a split second of peace and calm—then his back pain hit him "like a ton of bricks." He'd had a restless night, tossing and turning, trying to find a good position to ease the pain for more than a few moments, becoming more anxious about his sleeplessness by the minute—all on top of the pain itself.

As he made his way to the bathroom, he felt hopeless, frustrated, and anxious about the workday ahead. The pain was hard enough, but now with the third night in a row of poor sleep, he was coming unhinged. Peter noticed how angry he was at his physician, who couldn't find the right dose for his pain meds, and at himself for not being able to better tolerate the pain.

Being lost in the past and thinking about the day ahead affected how Peter felt in the present moment. We are all similarly lost much of the time. Our brain is constantly rehashing the past or rehearsing the future.

The truth is that the past is gone and the future isn't here yet. Of course we want to learn from the past and plan for the future, but not 24-7. Have you ever felt like your mind has a mind of its own? Welcome to the human brain! Mindfulness helps us take back what we want to focus on, namely the present moment, so that we aren't helplessly taken on a ride by our thoughts.

Because Peter suffers from chronic lower back pain he is caught in a typical version of rehashing and rehearsing "the pain story." When we are in pain—and especially when the pain has been there for a while—we not only experience the pain present in this moment but also immediately feel what happened around the pain in the past and what might happen in the future.

Each pain story has two parts:

1. the story of the past, and

2. the story of the future.

The story of the past is about how this pain came about: what was or wasn't done, what mistakes or oversights happened, and so on.

The story of the future often has two aspects:

1. Anticipation of the immediate future: how you will get ready for the tasks at hand and get through this day.

2. Worry about the broader future: what might happen if the pain doesn't get better or go away, or even gets worse.

Often the pain story leaves us to ruminate on: What could that mean to your professional life? Will you be able to keep working and earning money? Will you lose your current job? How will you be able to keep paying bills, including health insurance (if you have it) or all the other costs that come with suffering from a chronic condition? Or, what could you have done differently, even knowing that this kind of thinking leads nowhere?

What might the implications be for your personal life? Will your partner get sick of caring for you, being considerate all the time, and taking on more than their share of the home and family obligations? Will friends stop inviting you because you've declined so many invitations since the pain started? Will they get tired of your not being so fun and energetic anymore? Will you ever be able to hike/ski/run/lift more than five pounds (let alone your growing grandkids!) again?

In a moment of pain, a helpful reframe is that you are experiencing the physical pain that is here right now plus the emotional pain of the past *and* the future. That's quite a load to carry! No wonder we often feel completely overwhelmed, immobilized, and hopeless.

Current physical painful sensations + pain story of the past + pain story of the future = overwhelm

Carrying the pain story is like wearing a heavy backpack all the time even when it's not necessary.

How do we put the proverbial backpack down?

First, we must become aware of it.

Do you notice that you are upset about the past or worried about the future *in this moment*? If so, great! You have already done the most important step. You might wonder how being aware of what's happening can help—other than making you feel even worse, now that you have become aware of the story your mind is telling—but without this awareness you can't change anything.

You can only change what you are aware of.

That's step one. Step two is to actually put the backpack down. That is, we must practice putting down the stories we tell ourselves. We do so by internally saying, "Thank you, not now."

Then, we redirect our attention to something in the present moment that is more neutral, like the breath, for example, or the sensations of our feet on the ground. We are not trying to push the story away or stop it from arising in the first place. I'm sure you have tried that in the past. How did that work for you?

There is nothing wrong with thinking. Now, though, we have decided it's not the right time for this story to be listened to. We don't have to be angry at thinking or do anything about it. We're just refocusing our attention, like you would when you're absorbed in a work project and a colleague comes by with a question. We say something along the lines of "Hey, thanks for stopping by; please let me finish this up and then I'll get back to you."

Once we drop the story, the emotions that have been triggered by that story—the anger, the frustration, the sadness—will start to lessen their grip as we stop retriggering them with every repetition of the story. Don't get me wrong, this is not a onetime thing; you will have to do it over and over again!

We're then left with the actual sensation of the pain in this moment. What's that like right now, without being seen through the lens of the story? Often we realize that the pain itself isn't so bad in this moment, or at least it's way more tolerable than we thought.

Ana, who suffered from severe irritable bowel syndrome (IBS), came to class with a tense and tortured look on her face. She shared with us that she had a flare-up the previous night and was really scared about it. The last time this happened she ended up hospitalized and missed many days of work and income as a freelancer. The pain story had her firmly in its grip. We started with our meditation, and Ana was able to keep dropping the story over and over and return to the sensations of the breath, one moment at a time.

She started to calm down and unwind. After the meditation I asked Ana how her pain would feel to somebody who had never experienced it before. She paused and then laughed a little. "Oh dear," she said, "they would think they have an upset stomach."

When Peter remembered to drop the past and future stories for moments at a time, he realized that his back pain wasn't so bad, perhaps a 3 or 4 on a scale from 0 to 10: not nothing—but a level he could handle. He also felt tired, but he could see that if he didn't catastrophize about the future, spurred by events of the past, he was just that—tired. And he was able to take it one moment at a time to get through his day.

Practice: Writing reflection on the pain story

1. Write down your pain story of the past. What happened? How did this pain, injury, or disease start? What happened along the way? What didn't happen that you wish had happened? Was there bad luck? Were there mistakes, oversights, regrets? What emotions do you carry as a result of all this?

2. Do the same with the pain story of the future. What do you worry about with regard to your pain? What are you afraid could happen and what would be the consequences of that outcome? What emotions come up as you reflect on this possibility?

3. Now that you have brought these stories to the front of your awareness, you are more likely to notice them playing out—often as a result of a flare-up of the physical pain. At this point there is nothing you need to do with them. It's not about right or wrong or solving anything but rather about becoming aware of the flare-ups' effects as they play out in the present moment. The stories are like a colored lens that filters the present moment.

4. Ask yourself: In this moment do the stories ease the pain or exacerbate it?

5. If the stories exacerbate the pain, practice "dropping the story" one moment at a time by internally saying "Thank you, not now."

The pain story

Find a comfortable position.

Maybe make some small adjustments to allow the body to be as relaxed as possible right now.

Pause.

If you are in a seated position, feel your feet on the floor—simply feel the ground under your feet.

If you are lying down, feel any pressure of the bed, sofa, or floor against your heels.

Feel where your legs are in contact with the chair or the bed. Notice where there is touch and where there is none.

Do the same with your back. Notice if your back is touching a surface, like the back of a chair.

Now feel into what your hands are touching. Maybe your legs, maybe your other hand.

Pause.

Move your attention to where you can feel the breath in the body. Is it mostly at the chest or the belly? Can you feel the expansion and contraction as the breath rises and falls?

Pause.

Follow the rhythm of the breath. When you notice your attention moving elsewhere, gently bring it back to feeling the breath in this moment. Perhaps silently say "Thank you, not now" to the thoughts or distraction.

Pause.

Now notice if and where there are unpleasant or painful sensations in the body. Notice if it's in one area or several.

Pause.

As you feel into an area of physical pain, notice if there are thoughts about the past that are related to the pain. This can be the very recent past, as in the last hour or day, or the more distant past.

Pause.

Now notice any thoughts about the future related to the pain. What comes up?

Pause.

Are there emotions that come with those stories? Can you "drop" the story—even if just for a moment? Try saying to these emotions "Thank you, not now." And then come back to feeling a new breath.

Pause.

Or you can very lightly make a note to yourself: "This is the pain story" or "This is the past pain story" or "This is the future pain story." And then come back to the breath.

Pause.

Let any thoughts move into the background and simply keep the flow of the breath—moving in and moving out—in full awareness. Return to the breath every time the mind wanders.

"Thank you, not now."

Let yourself rest with the breath. There's no need to do anything, fix anything, change anything. If your attention is drawn to the unpleasant sensations in the body, you can also gently return it to where you most feel the breath in the body.

Pause.

In a few moments, our meditation will come to an end. Take time to transition, to open your eyes if you have them closed, and maybe stretch the body in any way it likes right now.

3

The Box We Call Pain

NO MATTER whether pain is acute or chronic, we want it to go away. We try to do something (anything!) about it, and if that isn't working, we attempt to block it out and avoid it as best as we can.

That reaction is natural, just a part of being human. No big surprise.

The mind relates to the pain by lumping everything related to this pain together in a box. Next, it slaps a big label on that box: "Pain." Then, it tries to shove the box out of the way to forget about it. It's just like what we do with boxes that we put in storage and label with just one word, like "summer" or "toys." After a few months or even years, we don't remember what exactly is in there because we haven't looked in it for a while.

However, this particular box—"Pain"—doesn't want to stay in the attic. It is in the way all the time. We try to go around it, push it to the side, maybe even drape a pretty cloth over it so that it's not just sitting there, ugly and in full sight.

Mindfulness invites us to reach toward this box and open it—with curiosity and even friendliness—to see what's truly in there, moment by moment. What we call pain is a complex, multidimensional phenomenon, made up of three main components: the physical or sensory, the emotional or affective, and the cognitive or analytical. Or put another way, it breaks down into the sensations we feel, the emotions the pain brings up, and how we think about the pain (the story around it). In the moment, though, we don't experience pain as a puzzle made of different pieces but rather as one solid image, which understandably often feels like way too much to handle.

Mindfulness can help break this big, overwhelming experience down into more manageable chunks. It will help us look at the three components one by one. The three areas are closely interconnected and influence each other, but they are not the same. When we work with them one at a time, they become smaller, manageable pieces.

Robert, a high-powered tech executive, came to me with excruciating back pain that was always present. The actual physical sensation was the biggest trigger for him. The guided meditation helped him explore the detailed sensations of the pain in his back. He realized that the area of his pain was only about the size of a quarter and that the rest of his body—99.9 percent—was actually pain free! This understanding flipped his perspective of the pain upside down. When Robert expanded his awareness to include the areas that were not in pain, the quality of his pain softened and his experience of the pain dropped considerably.

In contrast to his prior belief, Robert also reported that he had many moments during the day when he was completely pain free. But because these times weren't long, his mind had previously skipped over them, concluding that he was "always in pain." These two insights—the size of the area of the pain and the spurts of freedom from it—helped Robert relate to his pain in a new, more spacious way. The heavy box of pain had started to open and lighten its contents.

Practice: Working with thoughts, sensations, and emotions

1. Turn toward the pain with friendly curiosity (which might feel counterintuitive).

2. Bring awareness to the pain and ask yourself: In this particular moment, which of the three aspects of pain is the most active right now or contributes the most to the pain? Is it the physical pain, the emotions, or the story?

3. Focus on that part of your experience and allow the other two to move into the background.

4. Use your mindfulness and compassion tools, as described below, to focus on that part of the pain experience.

Strategies for each of the three components:

1. The physical sensation. Bring your awareness to the point where you feel the pain in the body. Where exactly is it? How big is it? What are the qualities of the pain? Are they, for example, sharp, dull, stabbing, throbbing, tearing, hot, tense, fluctuating? Do these characteristics change? Are they

there all the time or are they sometimes absent? Are they sometimes stronger, sometimes weaker? What about the rest of the body? Is one area painful or several? What areas are not in pain? How much of your body is not in pain?

2. The emotions. What emotions are present with the pain? For example, is there anxiety, anger, resistance, frustration, impatience, grief? Can you feel those in the body? And if so, where?

3. The pain story. What thoughts do you have around the pain? What meaning does the pain have in your life? These thoughts arise together with the emotions; for example: Will this ever go away? Why is this still here? What does that mean for my future?

With mindfulness and compassion practices we learn that we don't have to believe our own thoughts. We can let them move through our awareness like a flowing river. We learn not to take emotions personally; they will change and disappear if we don't reinforce them. And we learn to watch the experience of pain either from above, like an eagle-eye view, or in microdetail, homing in to deconstruct the concept of pain. We learn to have some compassion toward ourselves for the fact that we are in pain.

As was previously noted, the box called pain has three components—physical, emotional, and mental. Of those three, one often carries the load of the pain. More often than not, it is *not* the physical sensations. As a result, we can work with the emotions and pain story in particular ways that help the pain become a lot more manageable.

Physical sensations elicit emotions and thoughts. Emotions trigger thoughts that match the emotion; for example, when we feel anxious we will have anxious thoughts. Emotions themselves will also influence the level of pain; for example, fear or hopelessness will intensify the pain. Thoughts can also trigger emotions; for example, you may recall the accident where you were injured and anger and frustration arise.

In this meditation we explore the three components of pain and briefly spend some time with each. You can also choose to practice for a longer period with just the strongest component.

Opening the box of pain: exploring sensations, thoughts, and emotions

Let's begin.

Find a comfortable position.

Pause.

Maybe make some small adjustments to allow the body to be as relaxed as possible right now.

Pause.

If you are in a seated position, feel your feet on the floor—simply feel the ground under your feet.

If you are lying down, feel any pressure of the bed, sofa, or floor against your heels.

Feel where your legs are in contact with the chair or the bed. Notice where there is touch and where there is none. Simple.

Do the same with your back. Notice if your back is touching a surface, like the back of a chair.

Now feel into what your hands are touching. Maybe your legs, maybe the other hand.

Pause.

Now move your attention to where you can feel the breath in the body. Is it mostly at the chest or the belly? Can you feel the expansion and contraction as the breath rises and falls?

Pause.

Follow the rhythm of the breath. When you notice your attention moving elsewhere, gently bring it back to feeling the breath in this moment. Perhaps silently say "Thank you, not now" to the thoughts or the distraction.

Pause.

Now turn your awareness toward the pain. What sense of the pain is there in this moment? Where is it located? Is it in one area or more? If several, choose the one area that calls your attention the most. You choose: the strongest one—or not.

As you are holding this pain in awareness, notice what else is there that is related to the pain. Are there any emotions around the pain? How do you feel about the pain in this moment?

Pause.

What kind of thoughts are running through your mind as you pay attention to the pain? Thoughts about the past of this pain or maybe about the future—later today or tomorrow? Or even further out?

The physical sensations? The emotions? Or the story?

Pause.

Notice which one of three has the most charge to it—in this moment.

Pause.

For many people the story is what makes the pain so hard to tolerate. So let's start there.

Can you recognize a thought? How does a thought show up for you? Is it something you see—like written words or an image—or that you hear? Where do you become aware of thoughts? In your head? Above the head? Somewhere else in your body?

Can you allow thoughts—or thinking—to happen without getting lost in them or in the thought process? Can you *be aware* of thoughts instead of *being* the thoughts?

See if you find it useful to make a light mental note of thinking, as in, for example, saying in your mind, "Thinking, thinking" or "Future, future" or "Past, past." Is it possible to notice the beginning, middle, and end of a thought? At what point do you usually become aware of its existence?

Is it helpful to—firmly but gently—say "Thank you, not now" to the thought?

Pause.

Now allow the thoughts to be in the background, and let's turn our attention to emotions.

Are you aware of any emotions in this moment? If there are several, pick one to work with. If you aren't sure, come along anyway. We can work with a sense of "bland" or "numb" as an emotional state, too.

Pause.

Do you know what the emotion is? Is it, for example, fear, anger, frustration, overwhelm, regret, grief, sadness, loneliness? Or another emotion? Where do you feel it? Is it in the body or more in the head?

Where exactly is it? Can you bring awareness to where you experience the emotion the strongest and gently hold it there, without the need to change it or to make it go away?

See if you can allow the emotion to move in whichever way it needs to move. If you find it helpful, imagine breathing more space into that place.

Pause.

Address the emotion directly. For example, with fear: "Fear. This is fear. This is what fear feels like" or "This is what people feel like when they feel fear." Or "This is fear. This is a natural response for people in my situation."

Allow the words and the message to sink in. Avoid such phrases as "I'm anxious" or "I'm an anxious person." Don't make this emotion *who you are* but rather describe it as *an experience in this moment*, which comes and goes, like the weather.

Pause.

And now let the emotions move into the background, too, and turn to the actual physical sensations of the pain in this moment. If there is more than one area of pain, choose the one that feels the most important to work with right now.

Pause.

Where is the physical pain located right now?

What's its size?

What other characteristics do you notice? For example, is it dense, hot, searing, stabbing, throbbing, tearing, sharp, edgy, coarse, blunt? Does it have a color or a shape? Is it solid or fluctuating?

What else do you notice?

See if imagining breathing space into the pain is helpful for you. Simply infuse the painful area with breath and allow it to move and change as needed.

As best as you can, stay open and curious—or notice the contraction, the resistance. That is often part of the experience, to become aware of just how much we hate this and to notice how this resentment contributes to the pain.

Pause.

When you are ready, simply bring the awareness back to the breath and its sensations in the chest or the belly. If you like, take a few long, deep breaths and release the focus on the pain for now.

Pause.

When you are ready, open your eyes.

4

Self-Compassion for Pain

WHO AMONG US likes to be in pain?

Anyone? No?

So, when someone else is hurting, it's usually easy for us to be kind and compassionate toward them. But most of us aren't so great about being compassionate toward ourselves when *we* are the ones in pain.

The truth is that pain deserves compassion no matter whose pain it is, yours or mine!

Self-compassion teaches us to treat ourselves the way we would treat a good friend. Ask yourself: If a close friend suffers from pain, what would you say to make them more comfortable? "I'm so sorry you feel that way" or "The pain is really bad today, isn't it? Is there anything I can do for you?"

And what would you do? Maybe offer a hug or squeeze their hand if there isn't much to say? Do you let them know that you will be there no matter what?

Now imagine switching roles with your friend: How does it feel to be on the receiving end of kindness and compassion? It doesn't make the pain go away, but it makes a big difference in how we are able to live with the pain, doesn't it?

We know that receiving compassion from another person helps. It is less well-known that extending compassion toward *our own pain* also has a positive effect on the way we experience it. Do you treat yourself compassionately when the pain is bad? What do you actually say to yourself? What do you do? Do you try to downplay it—"Oh, it's not that bad"—or even deny that it's there? Do you chide yourself: "Toughen up, for goodness' sake!" or "Don't be such a whiner!"? Maybe your inner self-talk is much worse than this. I often hear from people that they internally beat themselves up and it often gets ugly.

If you treat a friend differently from how you treat yourself, then know that you are not alone in making this distinction: Research suggests that almost 80 percent of the US population are more compassionate toward others than to themselves. The good news is that self-compassion can be learned and strengthened!

The practice of mindfulness allows us to witness the pain and realize that while we are having an experience of pain it does not define us.

The practice of compassion for ourselves embraces *the part that is in pain* with kind attention. Compassion wishes for the pain to ease and go away but it doesn't depend on that outcome. That means compassion is still here even if the pain doesn't change.

One of the hardest parts of living with chronic pain is the loneliness that comes from the repeated sense that other people don't understand what we're going through. Acknowledging to ourselves—with caring and by witnessing—how hard this is and how alone we feel starts to calm the anxious and contracted nervous system. We begin to give ourselves what we wish from others: kindness, compassion, and presence.

Self-compassion has two main parts: kind awareness of the pain and the knowledge that suffering and pain are a part of life. We are not only talking about the physical pain here. There are many painful experiences that originate in the pain, like insomnia or the inability to do activities we used to be able to do. We learn to state the fact that this experience *is* hard or painful, the way a friend would, with kindness: "This is so hard right now!" or "This *is* painful!"

When we remember that experiencing pain is a part of being human and that many other people know the pain we are feeling, too, we begin to feel connected with our fellow travelers on this path we call human life. It helps us feel in solidarity with others who, past and present, are in the same situation and feel the same way. We are not alone!

Explore saying softly to yourself, "This is what it feels like to suffer from [insert ailment]" or "This is what it feels like to be so sleep deprived" or "This is what it feels like to be left behind."

Are there any shifts or changes?

Self-Compassion Is Not Self-Pity

When I ask people why they feel hesitant to be compassionate with themselves, they often say, "I don't want to throw a pity party." Or "I don't want other people to pity me, so why would I want to do it to myself?" They are confusing *self-compassion* with *self-pity*.

So, what's the difference?

Self-pity is the feeling that our circumstances are unfair and that other people don't struggle and suffer in the same way as we do. It tends to make us feel worse. We feel sorry for ourselves and (at least at times) want our friends to feel sorry for us. When other people pity us, it often gives us the icky feeling that they feel superior. After all, they don't have our struggles. It can feel like a little pat on the head, somewhat patronizing.

By contrast, compassion is knowing that we all suffer or struggle and that suffering is not a sign that there is something fundamentally wrong with you. It's not personal; it is universal. All humans will experience suffering and pain at some point. Instead of a patronizing pat on head, it's more like a kind hug or a squeeze of the hand. When someone acts compassionately, they're on your same level. No one is looking down on anyone.

Self-compassion expands the circle of beings that are included in the compassion, while self-pity includes exactly one person: Me!

Self-compassion isn't weak

To many, the idea of self-compassion feels weak. It can seem like giving yourself permission to stop trying and give up. These impressions came up time and again while I was working with Liam, a young combat veteran who served in the Iraq War. He learned to be "tough at all costs" and "a hero." Back in civilian life, however, he was suffering with severe chronic pain from explosion-related wounds as well as hearing loss and tinnitus (ringing in his ears).

The messages of toughness that were useful to him during his training and deployment did not seem to be helping him now. He came to a class for veterans that placed a particular focus on learning self-compassion. Each week, he showed up but always sat with his arms folded across his chest and never said a word. During the last class, he shared with the group how foreign this whole idea of self-compassion was to him. He said, "I came here because I was at my wit's end with the pain and my being so irritated and angry all the time. My wife basically threatened to leave me if I didn't do something. . . . Nobody ever told me that I could be kind to myself before." Liam then reported that in fact the class had helped him with the pain. He noticed that it wasn't so intense and said, "I'm no longer so furious about it all the time." Ignoring the pain or beating ourselves up internally just doesn't work. Why not be kind to ourselves instead?

Hugs for healing

Research shows that supportive touch from a friend or loved one, like a touch on the arm, squeeze of a hand, or hug changes the way we experience pain in that moment. This is definitely an important tool to have in our tool kit! Neurotransmitters like oxytocin and serotonin play an important role in these changes. Unfortunately we don't always have a friend around when we need this helpful internal biochemical cocktail. Here is a fascinating fact: Doing the same thing to ourselves has similar results.

Try it yourself: Hold a touch for a short period of time, 15 to 30 seconds, and notice how that feels. Is there a sense of relief, of letting go, of releasing? If so, then you're on the right track.

We are all wired a little differently, so what works for one person might do nothing for another. You can find out what works for you by giving it a try. Here are some examples of supportive touch:

a hand on the chest/heart area

both hands on the heart

one hand on the heart, one on the belly

a hand on the area that's in pain

squeezing or rubbing one forearm

giving yourself a hug, wrapping both arms around yourself

"secretly" holding your own hand while holding your hands in your lap (this is a favorite with many men who might otherwise feel sheepish about putting a hand on the heart)

Experiment with other touches that work for you.

This is available to you any time you struggle, and if you like, try it in combination with a phrase such as "This is a moment of pain. This is hard right now."

What to do when nothing helps

Sometimes the pain is so bad that it simply erases everything else. You are immobilized, can't think, can't talk, and most definitely can't meditate. In these moments, all you can do is give yourself a break, lie down, be still—maybe with a gentle hand on the heart. It might be too much to even say to yourself, "This is such a hard moment right now." But maybe you can move in the direction of that inner attitude of kindness toward this suffering, toward yourself.

And if you can't feel any self-compassion? Then see if you can have compassion for that—for the lack of compassion and the pain of that absence.

It sounds paradoxical, but it works.

Self-compassion for pain

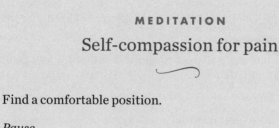

Find a comfortable position.

Pause.

Feel the connection the body has with the ground, the chair, or the bed.

Pause.

Is there any tension you can let go of? Release it and allow all other sensations to be present as best as you can.

Pause.

Connect with the breath. Take a few deep, slow breaths if that is helpful.

Pause.

Just breathe.

Pause.

Now place your attention on an area that is in pain or in discomfort right now. Feel what is here without overwhelming yourself. If it feels like too much, return the attention to the breath or even pause the meditation for a moment by opening your eyes and looking around.

Pause.

Put a hand on your chest or on the area that is in pain for support.

Find a phrase that acknowledges the truth of this pain—such as "This really hurts" or "This is a moment of pain"—and repeat it to yourself as softly and as kindly as possible. Keep repeating it for a minute or so, and see if you can let the truth of this statement sink in.

Long pause.

Now in your mind's eye, start to connect with others who are also in pain right now or even in the exact same pain, or who have ever felt this pain before. Maybe you feel them in a circle around you or at your back.

See if you want to make a statement about your pain in this light, like "This is what it feels like to experience [insert type of pain]." You could also say to yourself, "Feeling pain is a normal human experience. It is not wrong for me to feel this way."

Again, see if you can invite kindness into your statements and your internal voice. It's about *what* we say as well as *how* we say it.

Stay with this practice for a little while.

Long pause.

Now start to release all sentences and images and come back to just feeling the breath and the body.

Pause.

Take time to transition.

Open your eyes and close the meditation when you're ready.

PART 2

Making Peace

5

Ending the War with Your Body

"I HATE MY BODY." Amanda looked and sounded matter of fact when she said this to me, but her choice of words betrayed the intensity of her emotion. Amanda suffers from a severe form of psoriasis that affects her skin and joints. She added, "And my body behaves as if it hates me, too. It's like my body attacks me and I'm attacking it back."

Aren't you supposed to feel at home and at ease with your body, not wage war against it? Most of us believe that our body will function in a certain way. When it has stopped fulfilling that expectation, as when we experience chronic pain, we often feel as if our body has betrayed us.

Even before we have a chronic ailment, many of us treat our body like we would a car: It's supposed to work, and if it doesn't, then we'll bring it to the mechanic to be fixed. In my work as a physician, many patients would come in with this attitude. They would have loved to just leave their body with me for a couple of days until all defective parts had been replaced, the oil changed, and the brakes checked!

If the body hurts and can't be easily fixed—if we don't know exactly what is wrong—we get anxious or angry (or both) at our body and/or the doctors. In our minds, the body becomes the enemy. This attitude causes extra stress, pain, and tension in the mind and body, which in turn exacerbate our negative experience of the pain and life in general. It can feel like being trapped with our nemesis.

What does the war with your body look, feel, and sound like? Are you yelling at yourself or calling yourself names? Do you give yourself the silent treatment and withdraw loving attention? How do you feel when you are treating yourself harshly?

How would it make you feel if *another person* were treating you this way? Would you let them?

Mindfulness practitioners often talk about "befriending" or "hugging" your pain. For those with chronic pain, this suggestion typically elicits a look that plainly says, "You've got to be kidding me!" It's true, though. Befriending the pain is healing. But who can bridge that gap starting from a place of war? It's not realistic to move from aggression and hatred to being friends!

It might help to know that you can't force yourself to feel kind toward your body—nor toward anything else. We don't need to feel bad about it if *befriending* seems totally out of reach. We develop kindness and compassion over time, with intention, patience, and repetition.

Instead of pretending that there is no pain, mentally diminishing the severity of our symptoms, or falling into harsh self-talk, we can do something else—we can pay attention. We can acknowledge that, yes, there is pain. We don't have to like it in order to recognize it—and we can simultaneously hold feelings of resistance, hate, anger, disgust, or overwhelm that might be there along with the pain.

After acknowledging the pain, we may eventually *allow* the pain—because it is already there. This permission shifts our thinking from "I need to make the pain go away in order to feel in control" to "I'm taking back control by allowing the pain to be here—for right now."

Over time we might notice a softening in how we relate to the pain and to our body in general that can show up as *accepting* the pain in that moment, which doesn't mean that we give up on searching for new ways of healing. At the same time we learn that we are not defined by the pain—that we are so much more than just this pain. We might even *appreciate* the body for trying so hard to heal itself.

I call this practice "Taking the A-Train" (like the Duke Ellington jazz piece). We are moving from acknowledgment to allowance to acceptance to appreciation.

The A-Train

Acknowledge → Allow → Accept → Appreciate

At first this concept felt foreign to Amanda. We discussed why holding the body with more kindness and acceptance might be beneficial. Amanda feared that this was giving up—waving the white flag—and would lead to even more pain and disappointment. She understood, though, that her internal berating wasn't helpful and made her feel "wound up in tight knots." So she started to work on acknowledging the pain.

To start this process, Amanda would sit down for short periods of time, close her eyes, and turn toward the pain. This means feeling the pain as well as the mishmash of frustration, sadness, and other emotions related to her pain experience. She then softly repeated to herself: "This is a moment of pain" or "Here it is" or "This is what this pain feels like in *this* moment."

It is helpful to stay connected to the breath while doing this. Amanda reported that she would often become aware of a huge amount of muscle tension, some of which she was able to easily release, like dropping her hunched shoulders or releasing her clenched jaw. Over time this practice felt more natural and Amanda became calmer and more accepting toward her body. It simply felt better than being tense and upset about the pain all the time. Through acceptance, Amanda developed a new, healthier relationship with her body, which seemed to have an effect on her symptoms: Her skin and joints responded with less inflammation.

Using these awareness practices, Amanda learned to listen more closely to the body's needs, such as for rest or movement (e.g., changing her posture for more comfort). She said, "I realized that my body actually tries to communicate with me and that it doesn't want to be in pain either. I think it has become a kind of ally, so we can work together." She laughed and added, "I wouldn't go as far as to say that my body and I have become best buddies. But I would say that we now have a respectful and friendly working relationship, which is a huge positive change for me."

In this meditation I invite you to offer friendly wishes to the body. Initially this might feel quite foreign and even a little silly. We are trusting a basic rule of neuroplasticity, or changing your brain: Whatever we pay attention to will be experienced more often. With repetition, anything we do will feel more natural.

This practice is called a body scan. We'll move through the entire body, part by part, and 1) feel into each part, noticing what, if anything, is felt there and 2) wish each part happiness and calm by saying in our mind, "May you be happy and at ease." If you want to choose different words to express goodwill toward your body, that's OK, too. This well-wishing applies to all parts of the body, including those that are in pain, which need kind wishes the most.

If you suffer from insomnia—either having a hard time falling asleep or going back to sleep after waking up in the middle of the night—this practice will be especially helpful.

Kindness body scan

Let's begin.

Find a comfortable position.

Pause.

Maybe make some small adjustments to allow the body to be as relaxed as possible right now.

Pause.

If you are in a seated position, feel your feet on the floor—simply feel the ground under your feet.

If you are lying down, feel any pressure of the bed, sofa, or floor against your heels.

Feel where your legs are in contact with the chair or the bed. Just notice that—where there is touch and where there is none. Simple.

Do the same with your back. Notice if your back is touching something, like the back of the chair.

Feel into what your hands are touching right now. Maybe your legs, maybe the other hand.

Pause.

Now move your attention to the breath. Make these next few breaths a little longer and deeper if that feels OK for you, as if you could fill the whole body with breath.

Pause.

Let the breath flow naturally.

Pause.

As always, when you notice the attention moving somewhere else, gently bring it back to wherever you are in that particular moment. Maybe silently say "Thank you, not now" to the thoughts or the distraction.

Pause.

Now bring the attention into your feet. Simply feel whatever sensations are present there right now, like pressure against the heels or soles, or their temperature. You are not looking for anything in particular, just noticing what is already there. Sometimes there is nothing to feel, sometimes there is pain.

Can you notice it, without doing anything about it?

Pause.

And now, can you offer your feet some kind wishes? Try "May my feet be happy and at ease."

Pause.

Now move the awareness to your ankles and lower legs. Again, feel into what there is to feel. Then wish those parts well: "May my ankles and lower legs be happy and at ease."

Move on to your knees and upper legs. Check in with them.

Pause.

Then wish the knees and upper legs well.

Pause.

Now open your awareness to include the entire legs, from the toes up to the hip joints. Feel what it's like to have legs. Then wish those legs to be happy and at ease.

Pause.

Next pay attention to the lower trunk: the pelvis, the hips, and the lower belly. Notice any sensations there are to feel—or maybe notice the absence of sensations.

Pause.

In your own time, wish each of those body parts to be well, to be at ease.

Pause.

Let awareness be in the area of the whole belly, the area under the diaphragm, with all the internal organs that are inside the belly. Rest the awareness here. Do you notice any feelings expanding and contracting with the breath?

Pause.

Now offer friendliness to the belly, to the organs.

Pause.

Let go of the belly and move the awareness to your back, to the spine. What is there to feel today?

Pause.

Can you send an overall wish for ease and well-being to the entire spine?

Pause.

From here move on to the chest, the rib cage, the organs inside the chest. Feel the movement of the breath in the chest, expanding and contracting.

Pause.

Wish the chest and all the organs to be well, to be at ease.

Pause.

From here move the awareness all the way down to your wrists and hands. Feel and notice them. And then wish them well.

Pause.

Next are the forearms and the elbows. Check in and feel if there is anything to feel. There may or may not be.

Pause.

Wish them well with "May my forearms and elbows be happy and at ease."

Pause.

Feel the upper arms and shoulder joints with openness. Say "May my upper arms and shoulder joints be happy and at ease."

Pause.

Now open the awareness to include the whole length of the arms. Notice any sensations, like touch, position, or temperature. Then wish the arms well.

Pause.

Let go of the arms and move to the neck and shoulder area, where the big muscles are. What is there to feel in this moment?

Pause.

Say "May my shoulders and neck be happy and at ease."

Pause.

Move up to the head. Feel into the different parts of the head, the bones and the sense organs. Wish them well, wish them ease.

Pause.

And finally bring your awareness to the whole body. At the end of this body scan, feel the whole body. How are you now? How is your body feeling?

If it feels right, offer a wish to yourself: "May my whole body be happy and at ease. May I be happy and at ease."

Pause.

When you are ready, start to move the body, wiggling your fingers and toes. Maybe stretch the body in a way that feels good. End the practice in your own time.

6

Finding Your Internal Support Group

WHEN WE ARE in the thick of a personal struggle, it would seem that the last thing on our mind would be the pains and difficulties of other people. As it turns out, research shows that going through hardship and pain makes us more compassionate and empathetic to others over time, especially to people who are going through similar challenging experiences. We begin to see with more clarity and tenderness that others struggle, too, which in turn makes us feel less isolated and less prone to self-pity.

Think about the most compassionate person you know. What do you know about their life? Are you aware of their struggles and hardship? There is a good chance that this person has had their fair share of adversity and misfortune. As the saying goes, "What doesn't kill us makes us stronger"—and research suggests it also makes us *kinder*!

The philosopher Ken Wilber writes in his book *No Boundary* that "Suffering smashes to pieces the complacency of our normal fictions about reality and forces us to become alive in a special sense—to see carefully, to feel deeply, to touch ourselves and our worlds in ways we have heretofore avoided."

Mona told me that when her pain first started she felt like she had been cast out of a happy universe. She so longed to be back there. In the same way that a person who moves from light into darkness can't see anything at first, she felt utterly confused, alone, and lost. But like eyes adjust to the dark, at some point Mona realized that around her were other people with similar struggles. She was not alone. There was life and joy in her "new universe," but with a slightly different flavor, seasoned with a deep knowing about pain.

After some time of living with chronic pain, we might experience the lifting of a veil that was hiding another reality—one that we have been initiated into. We can suddenly identify pain in others, be it physical or emotional pain, and that familiarity releases a strong flow of compassion. Compassion is a combination of love and pain: When we bring spacious love to pain it turns into compassion. With compassion, pain is accompanied by love. Love is a strong positive emotion that—when experienced at the same time as pain—changes how we feel. Just like salt undeniably changes the flavor of the broth.

Studies show that people who have gone through a lot of adversity not only feel more compassion but are also willing to help and to give their time, money, and energy to those in need. It has long been known that people from a lower socioeconomic status score higher in empathy and compassion. The reason might be that in less-than-ideal circumstances people need to rely more on each other for support.

We can't overcome adversity alone. We need people to take care of us when we're sick—to cook, to take care of the dog, to drive us to doctor's appointments. After natural disasters like Superstorm Sandy (in 2012) and the 2011 earthquake and tsunami in Japan, the neighborhoods that rebounded the quickest were the ones that showed neighbors care for each other and could be counted on for support. We can't do it alone, but we can *get through it together*.

Helping others also counterbalances the dangerous tendency to self-isolate and head down a spiral of self-pity when you're in pain. You might recall from chapter 4 (page 47) that self-compassion and self-pity are quite different.

In self-pity, as with self-compassion, we acknowledge that what is happening to us is hard. But in self-pity, there is *no space to recognize another person's suffering.* All our attention contracts around us alone and how bad things are in our own world. Self-pity compounds the sense of isolation, the feeling that we've been singled out in misery and pain. It almost never inspires taking action or reaching out for help. It often leads to blaming others while waiting to be rescued, and it fosters a victim mentality.

Self-compassion is the same in that it also acknowledges that our experience is painful and challenging. We approach with care and compassion, the way we would with a dear friend who was struggling: "It is SO hard to feel that way!" But self-compassion doesn't collapse into isolation. Instead it opens into an acknowledgment that what is happening to us is part of being human.

Years ago, when a dear friend and colleague of mine was diagnosed with breast cancer, she shared that after the initial struggle with the question "Why me?" she realized that she needed to equally ask and reflect on the question "Why not me?"

"I know the numbers," she said. "I know how many women are diagnosed with breast cancer in their lifetime, so it's fair to ask, 'Why shouldn't it have been me?' I don't have an answer for that. This realization helps me to be kind to myself when I fall into the pit of self-pity."

Of course, there is nothing wrong with feeling self-pity, because it's a natural response in this kind of situation! But there are many, many other people who know exactly what you are feeling, because they have been in the same situation. This is not to diminish your pain and how bad it is—not at all! It extends the hand of connection that says, "Yes, me, too!" I get it. I get you. And yes, it is *that* bad.

It can be a big relief to learn that someone else has had the same experience, tragedy, or diagnosis. It doesn't change what you're experiencing, but it lifts the burden of being alone with your suffering. In a mysterious way, it softens the pain to know we are not alone and that there is nothing wrong with feeling the way we do. Hello, we're human! This recognition can be the tiny movement of the needle that moves the pain from unbearable to somewhat, somehow bearable.

Not good, not gone, but bearable.

This mix of self-compassion—of realizing that we are not alone and that we can't do it alone—and the shattering of the illusion of a perfect life or a perfect outcome is deeply transformative. We stop being so afraid of pain, be it our own pain or that of others. And we can start to be guided by Ram Dass's beautiful reminder that we are all just "walking each other home."

Shared humanity: calling up the internal support group

Find a comfortable position, either lying down or sitting in a chair. You can close your eyes or soften your gaze, whatever feels best to you in this moment.

Pause.

If you are sitting, place your feet on the floor and feel the solid ground under them. Can you feel the floor or carpet through your shoes or bare feet?

Pause.

Let your back be straight and upright if that is comfortable. You may lean against the back of the chair for support.

Allow the body to relax and loosen the jaw, the shoulders, the belly.

Pause.

Take a few deep, slow breaths, feeling the sensation of the breath in the body. Can you feel the breath in your chest or belly?

Release a little tension with every exhalation.

Pause.

Notice any feelings of pain, either physical or emotional. There's no need to be specific. In a broad sense, think about what you are carrying with this pain, this condition.

Pause.

See if you can acknowledge how hard and difficult it is to experience this pain, to have this pain, and to take care of the pain.

If it feels right, place a hand on your chest for extra support.

Pause.

If that feels right, say to yourself "This is hard" or "It's so tough to feel this way." Use words that you would find helpful to hear from a close friend who really understands what you're going through.

Pause.

Repeat these words a few times. When you listen to yourself saying these words, ask if you mean them. Does it feel good to hear these words? Or do you notice that you have a hard time accepting them?

Whatever your experience, it's OK. There is no right way or wrong way.

Pause.

Suffering from chronic pain often feels lonely. You might not know anybody else with the same condition, and most people you are close to won't understand what you're going through. But, in fact, countless people all over the world share what you feel. They know. They might even suffer from the very same condition.

In your mind's eye, invite all these people into your awareness—maybe as a small gathering of people, perhaps as a big group—to stand with you in solidarity.

I like to imagine them at my shoulders, with a line of people stretching back—and having my back. They get me. They know exactly how I feel. They are feeling the same pain or have felt it before.

Pause.

You are not alone—and you are not alone with this.

Pause.

Allow yourself to access a sense of connection with all these other people.

Pause.

Keep breathing, keep softening.

Pause.

Go at your own pace.

Pause.

And when you are ready, allow the image to dissolve. Take a few deep, long breaths. Move and stretch the body in any way that feels good. Open your eyes if you have them closed, then move on with your day.

7

Collecting Pearls

MINDFULNESS TEACHER and neuropsychologist Rick Hanson is fond of saying: "The mind is like Velcro for negative experiences and Teflon for positive experiences."

In other words, anything negative, stressful, or painful will be stuck in our memory, sticking out with greater strength. This is simply how our nervous system is wired. From a survival standpoint, it makes sense: If you learn quickly from a dangerous and threatening experience, you have a better chance of avoiding it or responding more effectively next time.

One day I was about to step into the street at a crosswalk when a car turning right almost ran into me. The driver didn't see me. Only my jumping back prevented me from being hit. My heart raced, and I was furious and scared! To this day I have a slight pang of fear when I am about to cross that street, even though that near miss happened years ago. My brain makes sure I have this place locked into my system as a danger zone.

So what about the positive? It turns out that good experiences don't have the same vital importance to our survival. Your life is not at stake if you don't remember the beautiful sunset or how amazing that fresh-out-of-the-oven bread smelled. Pleasant experiences appear and then disappear, like water running through a sieve. They don't easily leave a trace in our memory.

This results in a problem, however. Our brain keeps tabs on "how life is" through "implicit memory." This part of memory tracks the good, the bad, and the ugly, so to speak. Think of it as an internal shelf with cookie jars for each category. Depending on how full the individual jars are, implicit memory draws a conclusion about the state of your life, which generates a feeling or belief like the ones in the following examples:

> *"Life has its ups and downs but is still worth living"* or
>
> *"Life is a mix of difficult and wonderful"* or perhaps
>
> *"Life is one relentless struggle, one really hard thing after the next"* or
>
> *"Hardly any good things ever happen to me."*

Unfortunately, suffering from chronic pain is an ongoing process of adding to the jars labeled "Pain," "Difficult," "Hard," and "Fear" so much that they outweigh any pleasant events and moments that happen in the meantime, leading to a sense that there is no joy—or almost no joy—or happiness in life anymore.

Mindfulness practice can help with this challenge. One of the first mindfulness exercises we teach in a class is to eat a raisin—yes, just one raisin!—together. Nobody eats just one raisin, unless maybe you are two years old. We use all of our senses to explore the "raisin-ness" before we actually eat it. We share with each other what we discover. We look at the raisin, feel it, smell it, even listen to it before we pop it into our mouth and finally bite down. By that time everybody is totally engaged in the process and experiences, the explosion of flavor and texture. People often say, "That was the best raisin of my life!"

What is the takeaway message? If you pay full attention to something ordinary, it becomes extraordinary—and you will remember this. You just turned Teflon into Velcro in your memory! This kind of prolonged appreciation of one small thing is a powerful ongoing practice that, over time, can change how you experience life, regardless of the pain.

After a cosmetic procedure went wrong, Elizabeth suffered from chronic pain in her face. She became stuck in a cycle of blaming the aesthetician and herself for what happened. Her husband is understanding and patient, and they live in their dream house, which they built together years earlier. But the pain and her failed attempts at fixing it drained all the joy and pleasure from her life. When asked on any given day, she couldn't remember a single truly pleasant or joyful thing that happened that day or that week. I asked her to start a practice I call "collecting pearls." Here is how it works:

Practice: Collecting pearls

1. To set the intention to find pleasant and beautiful moments throughout the day, ask yourself: "If there were anything

pleasant or beautiful here right now, what would it be?"
Include all your senses in this exploration: What do you see,
hear, touch, smell, and taste? Also include the good company
of a friend or loved one, feeling cared for and loved, or
anything else you are grateful for.

2. Once you have found something pleasant or beautiful, bring
   your full attention to it for a few moments—take it all in, being
   aware that it is a joyful moment. Relish it, savor it. This is one
   pearl for you to add to your collection.

3. Imagine storing this experience and its memory, your pearl, for
   future use. Over time, you may think that you have a beautiful
   bowl that slowly fills with shining pearls. Some people like to
   even write these pearls down in a special notebook.

At first Elizabeth was skeptical. How would collecting these pearls help
with getting rid of her pain? But she was willing to give it a try, in large
part because her husband had repeatedly mentioned that it was hard
for him that she was so disconnected from their many blessings. She
decided to try this practice three times a day for a month. In the beginning, when Elizabeth tried to focus on something she used to enjoy she
only felt her familiar irritation. But her persistence paid off and she
started to feel little pangs of joy and even happiness when with friends,
when enjoying a nice meal, or when out in nature. By being aware of
these moments and through the practice of collecting them for her
bowl of pearls, she slowly started to feel a difference in her overall
well-being.

The pain in her face was still there but it didn't take up all the space in her experience. Elizabeth was able to feel that *yes*, there was the pain, *and* interwoven at the same time there were always moments of joy, connection, and gratitude.

The following meditation explores the experience of having feelings of pain or unpleasantness right next to feelings that are neutral or even pleasant. Instead of saying, "BUT there is pain . . ." which usually shuts the door on any further explorations, we say, "Yes, there is pain AND . . ." which allows for more than just the pain.

Yes, and . . .

Take a moment to find a comfortable position. Close your eyes if you'd like or just lower your gaze.

Pause.

Maybe move the body a little until it is just right for this moment.

Pause.

Feel into where the body has contact with the ground or with the chair, letting the body be held and supported by the ground or by the chair.

Pause.

And now connect with your breath. Notice where you can feel the breath in this moment. Is it at your nose, in your chest, in your belly? Simply feel the breath moving in and out.

Pause.

Would you say that your breath in this moment feels pleasant, unpleasant, or neutral?

As you bring awareness to different experiences, you can always keep a part of your awareness on these sensations of breathing. They are your anchor or handrail.

Pause.

Is there discomfort in your body right now?

   If so, is it in one part or in several areas? If several, choose the one area that is calling your attention the most. Either feel into this part of the body or stay at the edges, resting back with the breath.

   Now scan the body for an area where there is no discomfort, no pain. Can you feel absence of pain?

Pause.

Ask yourself: "What does that feel like?"

Pause.

Can you, maybe, find an area that feels pleasant? Perhaps your chest, with the breath, or maybe your eyes.

Pause.

If you find an area that feels pleasant, try to hold in mind both *discomfort* and *no discomfort* at the same time. Perhaps you can even hold *discomfort* and *comfort* at the same time, saying, "Yes, there is pain, AND there is no pain at the same time." Or "Yes, there is tension, AND there is no tension—or even relaxation—at the same time." Find words that work for you, feeling into the space that allows opposites—and everything in between—to be there at the same time.

We are not denying that there is pain, discomfort, or struggle. We are open to the possibility to say, "Yes . . . AND . . ."

Pause.

Take the time you need to end this practice, holding your experience and yourself with care and awareness.

Pause.

When you are ready, open your eyes and move on with your day.

PART 3

Handling
Big Emotions

8

The Dark Clouds of Depression

WHERE THERE IS PAIN, there may be depression—and vice versa—because these two conditions share important neuropathways. A vicious cycle often emerges in which pain worsens symptoms of depression, and the resulting depression worsens feelings of pain. If you find yourself in the middle of this cycle, how can you break it?

Chronic pain finds its way into all aspects of life: our work, our personal and family life, even our spiritual life. It often provokes existential questions like "Am I worthy?" "Am I a burden to others?" and "Who have I become?" We may have been highly active or athletic and now, because of the pain, are not—and it's not clear if we ever will be again. We naturally compare ourselves to others and come up short, painting a picture in our minds that we can't do as much, are not as strong, and can't be happy or peaceful in the way that people who don't have pain seem to be.

While studies suggest that up to 50 percent of people suffering from chronic pain have also experienced depression, it is also proven that regular mindfulness practice can mitigate depression. Researchers believe this happens in a few different ways.

One of the hallmarks of depression is negative and ruminating thoughts, such as "I'm useless" or "I am beyond help" or "This will only get worse from here." Mindfulness practice teaches us to see thoughts like these as *part of our experience,* like an itch or a scent, but *not who we are.* We don't need to believe every thought. We can learn to disengage from thoughts and rumination and return to the present moment with mindful acts such as feeling the feet on the floor or a soft breeze on the skin. Thoughts come and go, and negative thoughts don't need to trigger a downward spiral. Mindfulness practice helps us to become aware of—and eventually interrupt—automatic patterns within ourselves and in relationship to others.

Some of my students reported identifying tendencies to spiral. Matt described becoming aware that when he is in pain he tends to be more defensive toward any requests from family or colleagues, without having stopped to check if the request was reasonable or doable in that moment.

During a flare-up, Julie noticed that when her mood dropped, she stopped participating in group texts with her girlfriends, with whom she usually had daily, often fun exchanges.

And Kim recognized that she easily fell into all-or-nothing thinking that was activated through the pain-depression cycle, which resulted in her abandoning good eating, sleeping, and exercising routines when she was feeling low.

The boom-bust cycle is a well-known phenomenon with chronic health conditions: We tend to overdo it in times when there are few or no symptoms (boom), which often triggers a flare-up and then causes underdoing (bust). It's natural that we want to do more when we feel better, since it feels so amazing when the pain recedes. We may have renewed energy and euphoric thinking: "I'm finally better!" "This is the start of a new life!" Of course we then want to catch up on all the activities we had postponed or were missing out on. And then the bust feels even worse . . .

Mindfulness helps us see our reality more clearly—and with self-kindness. Increased awareness of our body and its needs can allow us to say no or take a break when we need to, instead of pushing through. Practicing mindfulness can help us become more attuned to ourselves and to what is needed in the present moment, which, for example, helped Kim to be more tuned in to her body and able to see when she started to speed up and instead make a conscious choice to take it easy.

By mindfully checking in with ourselves we can see when we need to slow down a bit and maybe cancel plans. Or the opposite: You might realize that, yes, having coffee with your friend this afternoon is doable and would be nice, even though you had a hard start of the day and thought you might need to leave work early to rest. A mindful pause and check-in worked for Matt—and helped him to not immediately jump to conclusions.

Mindfulness invites us to ask: "What is here right now?" and "What is the right thing to do right now?"

When pain is intense, it's often hard to be aware of anything outside of the pain. We have trouble seeing how to get through the moment at hand. With increased awareness, though, the world starts to open up again. We begin to notice the people around us, how we interact with them and they with us. We can make wiser choices about what does and doesn't work. It can create a stronger sense of connection and appreciation, which counters isolation—one of the main signals that chronic pain and depression are taking a toll.

With a little help from mindfulness practice, Julie found the courage to share with her friends how hard it was to reach out or respond when she felt low. Her friends responded with compassion—now, if they don't hear from Julie in a day and she isn't responding to the group chat, they reach out to her. That small act counterbalances some of Julie's thoughts from spinning out the idea that nobody cares and that she doesn't matter.

In summary, mindfulness helps with depression by allowing you to

1. Disempower ruminating and catastrophizing thoughts.

2. Reduce overwhelm through negative emotions.

3. Become realistic about what you can and can't do at any given time and be more OK with saying no.

4. Notice supportive people in your life and find new ways to relate and connect with them.

Safe and pain free in the body

Start by finding a comfortable position, or as comfortable as possible. Take a moment to check in with yourself with kindness to see if you can find a posture of more ease right now.

Pause.

Close your eyes if you wish. Feel the areas of contact the body has in this moment, like the feet touching the floor, or the bottom touching the seat of the chair or the couch. Feel into the stability and support of the surface beneath you.

Pause.

Now scan the body for an area that feels safe and that is not in pain. This area isn't causing tension or anxiety. If it isn't possible to find, look for an area that feels the safest and has a little less pain. Don't overthink this.

Pause.

How about your feet? Your hands? It could be your bottom on the chair. It could be your breath. Are any other areas safe?

Once you have found an area, anchor your attention there. This is the place to return to over and over, no matter where else the mind goes.

Pause.

Take your time. Allow yourself to slow down. Depression is mental pain. Real pain. And the mind has a tendency to focus on that pain. You can redirect your attention from this mental pain and the thoughts and stories that come with it, returning to the safe anchor in your body.

Pause.

There is no need to start arguing with your thoughts, no matter what they say. Thoughts are simply activity in your brain. Let them flow through your mind like a river.

Pause.

Notice thinking activity. If you find it helpful, say to the thoughts "Thank you, not now." And come back to the felt sense of your anchor, the place you've been directing your attention to. Really feel into the safety and stability of that anchor.

Pause.

If the attention goes into areas of pain in the body, practice the same redirection here. Firmly but kindly return the attention to your safe place. This will not make the pain go away, but it will leave the pain more in the background. Let your chosen anchor be in the foreground.

Pause.

What you are doing is not easy. Dealing with any kind of pain is hard—both physical and emotional pain at the same time can easily feel unbearable. And yet, here you are, working with it, being with it as best you can!

Can you give yourself some credit? For the courage and strength to simply show up here and to breathe and to feel it?

Pause.

When you are ready, let the meditation end in your own time and move on with your day.

9

The Fear of Making Grief Real

IN ALL MY YEARS working with people with chronic pain, I have found grief to be one of the most challenging feelings to address. Anger is understandable, as is fear, frustration, overwhelm, hopelessness, and so many other emotions that come up around pain, but grief is in a category by itself. Just considering grief feels like giving up the hope of getting better. Isn't that what grief is? Feeling one's losses? Isn't that automatically a prescription for feeling worse?

Tanesha, a physician in her forties who suffered from back pain after an accident and several surgeries, said that grieving would be like giving up hope that her back would heal. She would not only have to keep living with the pain but also consider the possibility that she would never go back to being a full-time surgeon, since her back couldn't handle the long hours in the operating room. She wasn't willing to accept that outcome. She said, "I'll fight this to the end; I'm not willing to give up."

The problem was that Tanesha kept fighting against the thing she felt was taking away her life—the pain—and against her sadness and a small inner voice that kept nudging her to face the facts. She was a physician, after all, and knew firsthand of so many patients' stories after back pain. It was confusing. What was the voice of hopelessness and depression and what was the voice of reason—of being real and learning to come to terms with what was happening?

We associate grief with the loss of something meaningful for us. Grief always involves coming to terms with the process of ending. It is itself a kind of death—of an identity we have been holding or our lens to the world (for example, "I'm the one who always took care of my sister").

Grief is a painful human feeling. There is nothing wrong with hurting this way.

Grief happens because we value what we lost or fear what we could lose for good. Grief is a form of honoring. We feel pain because we care.

Grief doesn't say anything about the future, only about our pain right now. We can be with this pain, one moment at a time.

Grief has its own rhythm, which is predictable in its unpredictability. It comes and goes and takes the time it takes.

We hold this with kindness and tenderness, as much as possible. It makes sense that grief is scary when we're managing an ongoing health condition. We hold some fear and doubt that our condition will not get better, that the pain will not go away. If we took the time to grieve what we've lost, it might make it all too real. It's terrifying to consider that we've lost our prior life, and we don't want to give in to that possibility. On top of that, the feeling of grief itself is so painful that most of us will go to some lengths to not feel it at all.

The problem with grief, as with any other emotion, is that if it's there, it's there, whether or not we allow ourselves to feel it. In psychology, there is the saying: "What we resist persists, but what we can feel we can heal."

When we don't take the time to recognize and really feel what's going on with us, it can fester. In fact, research suggests that unfelt grief can turn into depression.

Mindfulness practice allows us to

1. Recognize and name an emotion: "This is grief. This is what grief feels like."

2. Let the emotion simply be there, give it space, let it move through us in the present moment without getting lost in the story that comes with it.

3. Invite compassion for the fact that this hurts so much!

Trusting that she could use mindfulness to explore her emotional terrain, Tanesha was able to be less afraid of grief and sadness when those feelings did arise. She mustered up the courage to confide in a trusted friend with the grief she was feeling about a life she was losing. Her friend's compassionate listening made it possible for Tanesha to "have a good cry." She felt better and lighter afterward and realized that feeling and allowing grief is not the same as capitulating to the pain. She has since had several more "grief attacks," as she calls them, but it has become easier to let them happen.

Grief will naturally arise as you struggle with the unknown and uncertainties of a potentially chronic condition. The fact that you are feeling grief is not a confirmation that the pain will never go away! It's just a feeling. Keeping this in mind can help you allow grief to happen when it shows up. We can feel grief about a potential loss just as about a real loss. And we can learn to hold ourselves with kindness and tenderness when these intense feelings come up and acknowledge "It's so hard to feel this grief!"

The following meditation will help you when your grief is showing up more strongly. This practice is about being with the grief and allowing it to happen. Remember that grief is an emotion and it's not permanent, even though it might feel that way at times. Grief moves in waves. The more familiar you are with the patterns of your grief, the easier it becomes to stay afloat in the wave.

Being with grief

Find a posture that supports your body in this moment, maybe sitting or lying down. If you like, close your eyes and do a brief check-in to see if there is any tension you might be able to release.

Pause.

Connect with the breath wherever you feel it most prominently right now. Try taking a few long, deep breaths. Throughout this meditation, you can always return to the breath. The breath is an anchor for stability and support.

Pause.

Just breathe. Allow whatever feelings are here to be here. There might be sadness or frustration or the sense of grief. Or something else altogether.

There are no right or wrong feelings—just feelings. With strong feelings, sometimes it can be helpful to think of them as if they were someone else's feelings that you are keeping company for a while. Can you be with the feelings without trying to make them go away or turn them into something else?

Pause.

Can you name an emotion you are feeling right now? Softly naming the emotion to yourself can help you stay with the emotion. For instance, "sadness, this is sadness" or "grief, this is what grief feels like."

Pause.

How big are these feelings? As big as your chest? Do they fill the entire body? Even bigger?

Can you make space within you for whatever feelings need to be here in this moment? If at any point this feels too overwhelming, take a couple of deep breaths or open your eyes for a moment and look around. Emotions can be intense. Be kind to yourself and find the right balance between allowing the feelings and not being too overwhelmed.

Take your time.

Pause.

It's often helpful to put a hand (or both hands) on your chest when dealing with strong emotions, especially with sadness or grief. This signals support and connection to the body and helps to anchor and ground you.

Pause.

If tears come, that's OK, too. The body has its own language for feelings. Let it happen as best as you can and breathe with it.

In and out.

Allow whatever reactions show up to be here and to move through. Remember the image of the wave. It rises, it crests, and it falls. Surrender to this with awareness and with kindness.

You have a human body, and human bodies have emotions. Even feelings that seem as big as the universe will eventually change.

They rise, they crest, they fall. They are changing.

Grieving now doesn't say anything about how we will feel in the future. Right now, we can be with this pain, one moment at a time. We feel pain because we care. Hold this with kindness, with tenderness.

Feeling grief is a painful human feeling. There is nothing wrong with feeling this pain.

Pause.

In your own time let this meditation come to an end. Take all the time you need before opening your eyes and reentering your day.

10

Numbing Out

THREE MILLION AMERICAN CITIZENS and sixteen million people worldwide suffer from an opioid use disorder. In 2017, over seventy thousand people in the US died of a drug overdose, and more than 66 percent of those deaths involved an opioid.

Addiction is a complex topic and needs a lot more attention than this short chapter can give. The drive behind addiction is usually to numb pain. While many people drown out the challenging combo of emotional and physical pain—especially when there is also a history of trauma—with all kinds of substances, some have stumbled into opioid addiction after surgery during a time when physicians promoted the message that if you take a strong painkiller after surgery, you won't become addicted. Combine this casual attitude with loose regulations around prescribing opiates and you end up with a fateful combination for patients suffering from pain.

Fortunately, mindfulness can be effective in addressing symptoms of addiction. There are mindfulness classes explicitly designed for people in recovery from all types of addictions. For example, there is the eight-week Mindfulness-Based Relapse Prevention (MBRP) program; Craving to Quit, a mindfulness program to quit smoking; and Mindfulness-Based Eating Awareness Training (MB-EAT), to help with food addictions. They all work on the same principles of noticing and interrupting the craving cycle as are being introduced here.

I first met Omar in a mindfulness class I taught. He was a young man with a serious demeanor and a very slight limp who didn't share much in class but whose face would soften with kindness and compassion every time a class member shared something about a struggle they were going through. One day he stayed after class to ask a question, something he was too shy to ask in front of the group, and I learned about his story. After a snowboarding accident that shattered one of his legs, he had become addicted to painkillers. When new prescription rules restricted his access to the pills, he started buying them illegally, but he was always afraid that what he got was mixed with more dangerous substances. Omar feared that he might accidentally overdose, which happens to many people in his situation. He had read that mindfulness could help with addiction and had checked himself into a rehab program that uses mindfulness as one of its treatment modalities. That program had ended a few months prior, and he came to class to continue his journey of mindfulness practice and being sober.

Researchers have found that mindfulness practice targets brain regions that are implicated in addictive behavior—such as impulsivity, compulsiveness, reward seeking, and self-control. It also helps people regulate their emotions and behavior. One study showed that through regular mindfulness practice, participants' perceived stress and pain levels went down and their mood went up. The more the mood brightened, the more the cravings decreased. It makes sense that when we feel better, we also feel less in need of taking an addictive substance.

So how do we go about bringing mindfulness to addiction?

We start by using mindfulness like a flashlight that shines a beam of curiosity on craving and addictive behavior. The combination of curiosity and moment-by-moment awareness is quite powerful. *Curiosity* counterbalances *resistance*. Instead of pushing an experience like pain or a craving away, we can instead become curious about it: What is it like *right now*? Can we stay with whatever is happening in this moment?

Like they say in Alcoholics Anonymous (AA): You don't have to stay sober for the rest of your life; you only have to stay sober today, or rather—applying the mindfulness perspective—stay sober right now. Becoming curious about the experience, we can ask: What is this made of? What are the exact sensations?

When the craving begins, we can use curiosity to diffuse it. What makes it start? Is there a trigger? Is the trigger more physical or emotional?

What does the craving feel like? Where do you feel it? Does it have a pattern? What happens when you don't respond to it?

Are there pleasant sensations coming from the substance? Are there unpleasant sensations? How do they shift or change?

People find that cravings are made out of body sensations like tightness, restlessness, or a fast heartbeat. They can notice how their thinking quickens and hyperfocuses on what they believe will make the craving go away.

We can even be curious when we use medication or substances: What does that feel like? How does that make us feel? In a study on helping people quit smoking, participants were asked to be mindful while smoking. A lot of people discovered that they found the taste of the cigarette truly disgusting, which in turn helped them stop.

Shifting to curiosity from a *fear-based automatic reactive behavior pattern* is something neuroscientists can locate in patterns of brain activation and deactivation in a brain scan. They can see the deactivation of centers related to craving and compulsive behavior.

The MBRP program developed a powerful mindfulness practice called "urge surfing," through which people learn to stay with the rise and fall of an urge or impulse until it passes. Combining this technique with self-kindness and compassion made a huge difference for Omar and was the most powerful and lasting tool in his recovery. He had enrolled in a program with a multifaceted, supportive structure—which included individual therapy, group therapy, and short-term medication to help decrease the intensity of his withdrawal and cravings—that helped him be more present, moment by moment.

Omar learned that you can't get rid of a craving by trying to suppress it, argue with it, or ruminate or think about it. By giving it any attention, positive or negative, you give it power. A craving is like a wave that moves through the body, and our job is to learn to "surf that urge."

The saying "what we resist persists" applies here, too. But the opposite of "resisting" is not giving in; the opposite is allowing the urge to be what it is and riding it out until it subsides. And yes, when cravings increase, they often feel like they will never end until they're fulfilled, but that is only a part of the feeling, not the whole picture. We tell ourselves this story about the craving and with continued practice, we can change the narrative.

The following meditation can be done anytime and anywhere when you notice the start of an urge. You might want to do a couple of practice runs with "easy" urges first. Try to practice the full meditation for at least five breaths (or about a minute). Repeat as needed. In time, you will find your own way to practice urge surfing and gain a sense for how long and when to practice it.

Urge surfing

Start by finding a comfortable position, or as comfortable as possible. You can lie down for this meditation or sit in a chair. You can close your eyes or just soften your gaze, whatever feels best in this moment.

If you are sitting, feel the solid ground under your feet, maybe having a sense of the floor or the carpet through your shoes or bare feet.

Pause.

Let your back be straight and upright, if possible, or lean against the back of the chair for support.

Allow the body to relax, maybe loosen the jaw, the shoulders, the belly.

Pause.

Take a few deep, slow breaths and feel the sensations of the breath in the body, like the chest or the belly.

Release a little tension with every exhalation.

Pause.

A craving is a mix of thoughts about the urge and physical sensations, or what we call "the story." As you practice urge surfing, focus on the sensations but do not engage with the story. Don't try to suppress the story or argue with it—just let it be there, like background noise you don't like but can't do anything about right now.

Now notice where you feel the urge in your body. It can be in one place or several. If you'd like, do a brief scan through the body and check the places that are affected by the craving. Starting at the head, then proceeding to

the shoulders,

the arms,

the hands,

the chest,

the belly,

the legs,

the feet.

Focus on the area in the body where the craving feels the strongest. Turn toward it with curiosity, staying aware of the breath to help you steady your attention, like a handrail.

What exactly does it feel like? Tense? Hot? Throbbing? Tight? Tingling? There are many possible sensations. If it's helpful, silently name to yourself what you feel. Notice when the mind slips into thinking about the urge and simply come back to the actual sensation.

Pause.

Notice if the wave of the urge rises, stays steady, or falls. It might also ebb and flow.

Pause.

Repeat in other places in the body where you feel the urge.

Pause.

When you are ready, shift the attention back to the breath and end the practice in your own time.

11

Anger Is a Mixed Bag

CHRONIC PAIN is often accompanied by anger. And it makes sense. Anger is a natural response when things don't go our way, when life seems unfair or out of our control. And, no surprise, all those circumstances tend to come up with chronic pain. While ongoing anger is a common experience for people suffering from chronic pain, the reality is that anger makes the pain worse.

Many clients have described this correlation in different ways: Ralph, a man in his forties, said that anger was like a form of inflammation in his mind that worsened the inflammation of his arthritis: "It's like the heat of anger in my mind feeds the fire in my joints."

Gabriela said that anger made her shoulders and jaw tense up so badly that it often triggered migraines.

Pepe told me, "Feeling angry all the time just feels bad. But walking around like the world is out to get me and just wanting to kick or punch something feels horrible and is exhausting."

George, a vet who served and was injured during the Vietnam War, originally came to class for anger management. He had repeatedly threatened health-care providers and was known to start fights—especially when drunk. It turned out that George also suffered from multiple forms of chronic pain, some related to war injuries, some just because of his age.

"This anger is a beast, I tell you," George said. "I'm feeling OK and then something happens or somebody says something and—*bam!*—before I know it, I'm already yelling. And then I'm fuming for days afterward. I feel horrible that I can't control myself."

I asked George if the anger influenced his pain levels.

"Now that you say it, Doc, I think it does. Big-time actually. I'm getting so tense in my shoulders and neck that it makes the neck pain worse and I often get bad headaches, too."

This realization motivated George to dive fully into learning mindfulness. When he and I chatted a few months after the class he shared with me that he is much more able to control his anger. He said, "It's weird but I can now actually feel the anger as it's stewing in me and I can then go for a walk or hang up the phone. Before I didn't even know the anger was there until I blew up. Now I notice that my hands and my face are getting warm and that's a sign for me that I need to move away from the situation." When I asked him about his pain levels he shared that he noticed that his headaches have become less frequent. "The anger is like fire in my body, and my head and joints don't like that at all. So not letting the anger get so big and out of control seems to be good for my body, too."

Anger gives us a sense of power when we we're not in control. Anger can energize us to take action; for example, to speak up with a health-care provider who is not giving us adequate attention, who is not really hearing us.

However, anger often distracts from the feelings that lie behind it—like fear, grief, and hopelessness. Anger is often the "hard" emotion in front of those "soft" ones. Depending on your upbringing you may have learned that it's not OK to express anger—or to have it at all. To be angry may have been looked down upon as a deep flaw in your character. This conditioning makes it difficult to investigate the feelings behind our anger in any meaningful way.

Mindfulness can help us correct course. One of the first things we may discover—as Ralph, Gabriela, and Pepe did—is that anger usually makes pain worse. Anger puts the body in a heightened state of alarm in order to ready the body to fight or flee. In an acute state of anger, pain *can* be suppressed to allow our focus to shift to the object of our anger—but not if the pain is chronic and we can't suppress it for long. This moment of suppressed pain is a numbing spike, not a sustained condition. When we move past the acute moment of anger, the pain is still there . . . and the anger may rev up again at any moment. It's easy for the anger to turn chronic with chronic pain.

When the anger becomes chronic, it manifests as resentment or bitterness. It's like a festering wound that prevents us from moving forward to adapt to new circumstances; it insists that our life should be different, despite evidence that life is what it is, and we can't go back and change our circumstances. There is a saying that anger is like picking up a hot coal to throw at another person. We can't touch it without being affected by it.

In our body anger manifests as active muscles, increased heart rate and blood pressure, and a release of adrenaline. The body prepares to fight the originator of the pain. Our attention narrows and becomes locked in on the target of the anger. Other priorities are pushed aside and forgotten. The body (and mind) pays a price for this highly charged energy, especially if it is sustained over time. That's why we call anger a mixed bag.

Psychology teaches us that anger has two basic directions: in and out. People who turn their anger *in* turn it against themselves, for example, in the form of self-judgment, self-berating, or even self-harming. Many psychologists believe that depression is a form of anger directed against the self.

When anger is directed *in* toward the pain it shows up in the form of hate—hating the pain or hating the body that causes the pain. It may also appear as a harsh inner voice that berates you for having made mistakes in preventing or treating the pain. You may scold your body for being too weak to heal. That inner voice can sound like: "I hate this damn useless body of mine.... Why didn't I get that checked out sooner...? Why did I ride my bike on that crazy steep mountain...? I HATE this pain; it never leaves me alone."

Then there is the acting *out* of anger; for example, using an aggressive tone of voice, choosing harsh words, or carrying out harmful acts against others. This often shows up when dealing with doctors, health insurance companies, or inconsiderate family members—anyone who made any mistake at any point—even God for letting you be in such pain.

In both the inner-directed and the outer-directed anger, we're avoiding the actual emotion of anger. In the first case, as we work hard to suppress any outward motion of anger, we are often not aware of the angry self-talk. In the second case, we may have a rapid, automatic, and thoughtless reaction while hoping that by expressing the anger we'll also get rid of it. Instead, this often sets off a chain reaction.

Let's be clear: It's OK to feel anger. Being made to feel guilty about anger brings no relief. What you feel is not your responsibility, but what you do with it is—and what counts! As with all emotions, our relationship with it determines whether it is harmful or helpful.

In mindfulness practice, we learn to make space for ALL emotions, including anger. We learn that emotions are just energy moving through us. (Have you ever noticed that the word *emotion* has the word *motion* in it?) The first step is to become aware of when we're feeling a particular emotion.

Each of us will experience anger a little differently. For some of us, it is a physical experience: the tightening of the jaw, a pulsing in the temples, or hot hands. For others anger can be experienced mentally, like having racing thoughts that have a sharp edge to them or that are accompanied by strong or even violent images.

Once you know where you experience anger, turn toward this experience with curiosity and openness. You don't have to like the anger, but you can simply acknowledge it: "Yes, there is anger. And this is what is feels like right now." It can be helpful to imagine creating some space around the anger, like a large corral for a wild horse.

Can you be specific about the sensations you feel without getting lost in the story of who did what to whom? Let the sensations be there;

observe them. If it's helpful, validate them: "This is what anger feels like" or "This is a moment of anger" or "There is a lot of anger here right now." You could also use "A part of me is very angry right now."

This practice is not to make the anger go away but to get to know it better so that we can work to not turn it against ourselves or another person when it arises.

As we practice, we learn the following:

1. Anger is one of the many feelings we have.

2. Anger comes and goes.

3. We can feel anger and what it would be like to act on it without actually doing that.

4. We can listen to anger as a consultant: We listen to what it has to say but we decide if we want or need to act on it.

5. Behind the protection of anger, there are often other feelings, like sadness or fear, that are equally justified and also need our acknowledgment.

Safely exploring anger

Find a comfortable position, or as comfortable as possible.

Pause.

Take a moment to connect with the ground under your feet or the chair or whatever surface your body is resting on.

Pause.

Let yourself feel the support of that ground. If you'd like, connect with the feeling of the breath. The breath can be an anchor to help you through challenging moments.

Pause.

How is the body is feeling right now? Maybe tired, maybe tense, maybe achy, maybe restless, maybe kind of OK, maybe all of the above or something completely different.

Pause.

As best as you can, allow whatever is already here to be here.

We are about to explore the emotion of anger. If at any time it becomes too intense for you, then pause for as long as you need. It isn't a problem. You can come back to focus on the breath or can open your eyes, look around, take in your surroundings, and resume when you feel ready.

Pause.

Can you allow openness and even curiosity as we explore this topic? Maybe you feel anger in this moment, maybe you don't. Check if there is anger in your system.

How do you know you are angry?

What in your system tells you there is anger?

Where do you check and how do you notice?

Pause.

As you bring awareness to any sensations of anger you've found, can you *become aware* of the anger instead of *being* the anger? Maybe you can name for yourself what is going on: "This is what anger feels like" or "There is a lot of anger here right now."

Pause.

Name it. Breathe with it as best as you can. Give it as much space as possible. Imagine creating a wide corral around the anger, like a wild, upset horse, not trying to wrestle it down but giving it space to express itself. Remember the breath, using it like a handrail to guide you to the present moment.

Pause.

If you need to, toggle back and forth between the breath and the feeling of anger.

Pause.

If you notice that you are caught in the story of who did what to whom, gently but firmly turn your attention back to the actual feeling of anger.

Pause.

Maybe notice the effect that the retelling of the story has on the anger. Does it make it better; does it make it worse?

What happens to anger as you stay with it without the urge to make it go away?

Does it change into something else?

Pause.

If the anger gives way to another emotion, welcome it, name it, and give it space.

Pause.

Repeat as necessary if other emotions arise.

Pause.

And now, when you are ready, release the focus on whatever emotion or emotions might be present right now and come back either to just the breath or to the whole body and the breath.

Pause.

Open your eyes in your own time and continue with your day.

12

Freeing Yourself from the Prison of Resentment

FOR A YEAR, Sabrina received the wrong diagnosis and treatment for her chronic progressive illness, which left her with permanent damage to her body and ongoing pain. She used to be extremely angry about it and thought a lot about revenge.

At some point, that changed.

Sabrina said, "I realized that the revenge I was holding on to wouldn't give me back my health, but that I kept torturing myself with it and it kept me up at night. The pain was bad enough in itself. I didn't want to keep carrying this hatred in my heart around with me anymore."

Forgiveness is a practice of freeing your own heart from the prison of pain and resentment. Forgiveness doesn't mean you have to condone what happened or agree with it. You don't even have to like it—not at all. It's a realization that holding on to what happened is in itself painful.

Meditation teacher Jack Kornfield likes to say, "Forgiveness is giving up all hope for a better past." Angrily holding on to what happened is painful and can easily turn into bitterness. That's not a place where we want to live our life.

We practice forgiveness understanding that we have all betrayed or harmed someone—out of our pain, fear, anger, or confusion—whether we know it or not, just as we have been betrayed and harmed by others. For example, we make a wrong assumption about why somebody did or said something and then we lash out. Or in a moment of acting or speaking we don't think about what our actions might mean to the other person. Not to be glib about it, but it's simply part of the human condition. Nobody is spared.

Do you feel that you're holding anger or resentment against somebody, related to your pain? It might be the person who caused your accident; it might be the surgeon who did the first operation on your back—or the second or third; it might be your sister-in-law, who always treats you like you're just pretending you're in pain so that you can sit and rest while everybody else is helping around the house.

Maybe—and this is usually the hardest part—you feel like you can't forgive *yourself* for something, like seeking medical help so late, or trusting in your doctor's/mother's/friend's advice, or smoking or eating too much of one thing or too little of another.

Whatever the cause or the content, not being able to forgive hurts. Sure, anger can feel good at times. In the beginning, it can give us energy to speak up or to make a change, but then what? What does it feel like to be caught up in anger that is way past its best-by date?

We can use our mindfulness practice to turn toward these feelings and notice: What does it feel like to keep holding on? What emotions come up in that moment? Does this influence your pain levels in any way? Jack Kornfield asks us to "sense the suffering that comes with the inability to forgive."

While in his yard, Harry slipped on the deck and broke his hip, which led to several surgeries and wounds that became infected. In the end, he had to live with a permanently limited range of motion in his right hip and nerve pain on the right side of his pelvis. After years of litigation, Harry successfully sued the company that built the deck. His lawyer was pleased that all of Harry's medical expenses were paid for by the company on top of a substantial amount of personal injury compensation. Through all those years, Harry had nursed the hope that once he won the lawsuit—once the company apologized and were made to pay—he would feel a sense of redemption and would finally be able to let go and move on with his life.

Indeed, he did feel relief and was grateful for having most of his living expenses covered for many years to come, but his anger and resentment didn't go away. He found himself picturing the CEO of the company being on vacation in a beautiful place and having no idea of the amount of pain and suffering Harry was in BECAUSE OF HIS ROTTEN DECK! When his pastor suggested to Harry that he practice forgiveness for the company and its boss, Harry scoffed. Then the pastor told him a story:

Two prisoners of war ran into each other a couple of years after they were released. One asked the other, "Have you forgiven our captors yet?" The other one answered, "No, I will never forgive them!" To which the first replied, "So they still have you in prison!"

That got Harry's attention. He realized how much he was still a prisoner to what had happened, and he wanted to free himself. When I met Harry a few years after this episode, he said, "I had already done everything I could to make the [physical] pain better; there wasn't anything else I could do. But I could start to work on my mind—to learn to forgive, to release that big pain and truly move on."

Forgiveness takes time. It doesn't happen overnight. We cannot simply decide to forgive and think that will take care of it. For most of us, forgiveness is a slow process that takes place gradually, often over years. So please be patient with yourself! The first step is to realize that to forgive might be a good idea—at least theoretically—even if it feels like you could never do it.

Start by setting the intention to learn to forgive. You can practice this meditation regularly or use the steps or words as needed throughout the day. Some people use prayer, some use journaling, and some talk to friends or a therapist to help them gain more clarity about where and how they are stuck. No matter what your approach is, sustained intention over time, put into practice in small steps, will result in change.

Forgiveness is traditionally taught in three iterations.

1. We ask for forgiveness from the people we have harmed or hurt.

2. We practice forgiveness for the people who have harmed or hurt us.

3. We practice forgiveness for ourselves for having harmed or hurt ourselves.

Forgiveness

Take a moment to settle into your practice by finding a supportive posture, maybe by closing the eyes or taking a few long, deep breaths.

Pause.

Arrive into this moment, into this body as best as you can. If you'd like, place a hand on your chest as a gesture of support and presence.

Pause.

Remember that we are not trying to make ourselves feel anything. We are simply inclining the mind and heart in the direction of forgiveness. You might feel emotions and you might not. Whatever is arising is OK, and we welcome it as best we can into this moment, without pushing it away or holding on to it.

You are in charge. Go at your own pace.

Pause.

Let yourself feel the barriers, the pain, and the many emotions you are holding by not forgiving—not forgiving others, not forgiving yourself.

Is an intention arising to forgive, to learn to forgive?

Pause.

Let's begin by asking for forgiveness from those we have hurt or harmed. This can be in regard to your pain or more generally. Go with what feels right to you.

Say to yourself: "There are many ways I have harmed or hurt another, betrayed their trust, knowingly or unknowingly, through my own pain, anger, fear, and confusion."

Pause.
Let yourself remember the many ways, all the occasions. Let yourself open to the pain, feel the sorrow and regret. You might feel your readiness to finally let go and to ask for forgiveness.

Say: "I ask for your forgiveness. Please forgive me."

Pause.

Say: "I ask for your forgiveness. Please forgive me."

Now release this part of the practice by taking a few long breaths, feeling into the shoulders and neck.

Pause.

We are now moving to forgiveness for those who have hurt or harmed us.

Say to yourself: "There are many ways I have been harmed or hurt by another, ways they have betrayed my trust, knowingly or unknowingly, through their own pain, anger, fear, and confusion."

Pause

Let yourself remember these many ways, in regard to your pain or more generally. Feel the ways you have been hurt as well as the pain of still holding this pain and resentment. Feel the potential release that could come from letting go and forgiving. To the extent that you are ready, offer forgiveness: "I forgive you. I release you."

"I forgive you. I release you."

Or "I am setting the intention to forgive you or to learn to forgive you." Use the language that makes the most sense to you right now.

Pause.

Take another couple of deep breaths to release this part of the meditation and turn toward the last part, forgiving yourself.

Say to yourself: "There are many ways I have harmed or hurt myself, many ways I have betrayed myself, knowingly or unknowingly, through my pain, anger, fear, and confusion."

Pause.

Let yourself feel the many ways you have betrayed and harmed yourself, in regard to your pain or in general.

Let yourself feel the sorrow and regret; let yourself feel the preciousness of your body and mind. Remember that you are not the same person anymore, that you have grown and changed. You didn't know what you know now. Or you knew but couldn't quite practice it yet.

Pause.

Feel into the release that might come from forgiving yourself.

Pause.

To the extent that you are ready, offer yourself forgiveness: "I forgive myself. I release the pain of not forgiving myself."

"I forgive myself. I release the pain of not forgiving myself."

Or "I am setting the intention to forgive myself—or to learn to forgive myself." Use the language that makes the most sense to you right now.

Pause.

And when you are ready, slowly release this practice of forgiveness. Come back to your breath for a few minutes or feel the whole body again.

Pause.

Take your time to end this meditation and move on with your day.

PART 4

The Pain of Connecting and Disconnecting

13

Dealing with Ignorance

PAIN IS MOSTLY INVISIBLE. It's not necessarily obvious to others who look at us that we are experiencing ongoing pain. And many of us will go to great lengths to cover up just how much pain we are in. We might hide it with strangers or with colleagues in order to be seen as capable; we may feel at risk of losing our job—if we are still able to work, that is.

We want to be seen—and treated!—as a "normal," pain-free person. None of us want to be pitied or tiptoed around. We also don't want others to make assumptions about how we feel or what we can or cannot do. Interacting with other people can be tricky and awkward under the best circumstances. Chronic pain can take tricky and awkward to new levels!

If your pain condition has been around for a while, most if not all of the following remarks will be all too familiar:

You don't seem sick!

My aunt had the same thing and she was cured by . . .

Everything happens for a reason.

God doesn't give us more than we can handle.

It's all in your head.

If you would just exercise/sleep more/eat better, you'd feel a lot better.

Have you tried . . . ?

My massage therapist helped me a lot; you should try her.

Really, it can't hurt that much . . .

I think you're just being lazy; everyone has pain.

You're too young to be so sick or in so much pain.

We hear statements like this—from the mildly suggestive and clueless to the harsh and vindictive—from family members and friends, at doctors' offices, at work, and at social gatherings. Most often the person making the remark doesn't mean anything negative by it and likely wants to be helpful, but that doesn't keep it from being hurtful, especially when you've heard it many times before. These remarks often imply that the other person knows better than you and that what you're doing or feeling is wrong.

In a conversation I was having with Martin, a young man with rheumatoid arthritis among other autoimmune issues, it wasn't hard to see the toll that these types of comments take. He said, "I can't even count the times I've heard *You are too young to be in that much pain. . . . You look too healthy. . . . Surely it can't be that bad.* I know that I look muscular, and people always assume that I can't be in pain or that if I say I can't lift this or I can't do that, then I must be lying. I'm so tired of feeling I have to justify myself all the time. As if I don't also hate that I'm not be able to do all those things I feel I should be able to do."

Repeated comments that are dismissive, alienating, invalidating, and overall hurtful come about from our being part of a marginalized group and are known as *microaggressions*. Originally coined around race, the term has been expanded to other groups—like religious minorities, LGBTQ+ communities, or people of size—who are targets of discrimination.

Microaggressions are characterized by their accumulating negative effect on the receiver. A single remark, while hurtful, can usually be dealt with—but repeatedly being subject to derogative stereotypes is draining and has a lasting effect on the nervous system. The result has been poignantly described as a "death by a thousand paper cuts." The erosion is even worse for people with chronic pain who are also part of other targeted groups.

Maria, a third-generation Latina from Los Angeles, suffers from severe endometriosis. She says, "I don't sleep well because of the pain and have only short windows during the day when I can do 'normal' things. I often have to cancel appointments because I'm too tired or in too much pain. People don't get it that I'm sick. Sometimes I just see in their eyes that they think *Oh, another lazy Latina—mañana, mañana!* I have even had it said to my face: 'I wish you people would show up if you say you're going to!' You people!"

These remarks often emerge as a result of others being uninformed, making assumptions, and feeling helpless in the face of someone in pain. When someone dispenses advice (Person A) or assumes they know what another person (Person B) is feeling or going through, it can lessen their own discomfort and make them feel better. This is an extremely common, often automatic response, so much so that Person A rarely thinks about it until Person B looks hurt or closes up. Then Person A feels guilty and easily gets defensive because, after all, that was not what they meant! And why does Person B need to be so sensitive?!

What can you do about hurtful remarks and microaggressions?

The consensus view is to pick your battles. Constantly having to educate people is exhausting. For example, letting people know that you are not lazy because you need to take the elevator instead of the stairs. Or that taking a nap or getting a good night's sleep is not the solution for the fatigue associated with your chronic pain. Or that your recent weight gain is not from binge eating, junk food, or lack of exercise, but because it's a side effect of your steroid medication.

When you have been hurt and must decide which battles to pick, mindfulness and self-compassion are great tools to take care of yourself. Mindfulness helps you become aware when a microaggression has happened and to label it as such. Remember that labeling an experience as what it is allows us to step back a little from identifying with it: to be *aware* of an experience instead of *being* the experience!

Then, we can offer ourselves self-compassion for just having been hurt: "It's so painful to be on the receiving end of such a remark (again!)." Remind yourself that the remark says way more about the other person and their mental state than about you. These two steps help the nervous system to calm down so that we can decide if we need to fight this particular battle now, respond later, or let it slide this time.

Sometimes we need to take time to talk it through with a friend or tribe member (see page 165). Receiving the compassion and understanding of somebody who understands how annoying and hurtful these remarks are can be helpful. We have to be careful, however, that these conversations don't fuel the fire of anger (see page 121) or cement a sense of "us" versus "them."

If you're the one receiving the insensitive remark . . .
Here are some helpful things to think about when considering whether to speak up (modeled on suggestions by psychologist Kevin L. Nadal in his *Guide to Responding to Microaggressions*):

> *How much does it matter to me that this person understands why what they said or did was hurtful?*
>
> *If I speak up, can I expect the person to listen and be open to what I have to say, or will they get defensive and hide behind "That's not what I meant" or "You are too sensitive"?*
>
> *If I speak up, how will this affect my relationship to the person (family member, coworker, doctor, etc.)?*
>
> *If I don't speak up, will I regret it?*

If you're the one having made the insensitive remark . . .
What's the best way to respond when we have accidentally hurt or offended someone, or dismissed their pain?

> *Listen and don't defend yourself. Try to learn why what you said or did was offensive.*
>
> *Don't hide behind your good intentions. The other person just told you that your remark made them uncomfortable: Can you stay open for a learning opportunity and acknowledge that there is a difference between intention and impact? You are not a bad person; you just didn't know! Next time you will know better.*
>
> *Apologizing is good, but listening and trying to understand is even more important!*

In a nutshell: Validate, get curious, try to learn what's really going on, and don't give advice.

Use the following meditation when you are processing a hurtful remark. Once it has become familiar, you can shorten or adapt it to use during the conversation itself by focusing on just one phrase as a kind of mantra.

Dealing with hurtful remarks

Start by finding a comfortable position, or as comfortable as possible.

Pause.

Take a moment to connect with the ground under your feet or the chair or whatever your body is resting on. Let yourself feel the support of that surface.

Pause.

Connect with the feeling of the breath.

Pause.

How is the body feeling right now?

Pause.

If you'd like, place a hand on your chest or another part of the body as a gesture of kindness and support.

Pause.

Now let yourself feel the impact the remark had on you, but don't get lost in the story and, if it arises, the angry back-and-forth in your mind.

Stay with the sensations in your body. Where do you feel the impact? In your chest? Your shoulders? Your belly? Your arms?

Pause.

The first response is often anger or another fierce emotion. Remember that anger is a protector that helps us set boundaries. Whatever emotion you're feeling, let it be there. If it is anger, it might need more space. Can you invite openness into your experience? Try it with the breath, as if you could breathe more space into and around the anger.

We say that anger often needs a big pasture to let the energy it's holding move through, like a wild horse needs a big pasture.

Pause.

You can name the emotion: "Anger" or whatever the emotion is. Welcome it as best you can.

Pause.

Anger might stay as it is, and it might start shifting into something else: Sadness? Grief? Hopelessness? Loneliness?

Whatever arises, can you stay gentle with it? Breathe with it. Remember that it's in the nature of emotions to move. Allow change to happen.

Pause.

Validate what you feel by softly naming it, if that feels right.

Pause.

Start to also validate your hurt. Try saying "It's so hard to feel this!" or "This is a difficult moment."

Pause.

Softly repeat some loving wishes to yourself:

"May I be gentle with myself."

"May I feel safe and protected from internal and external harm."

"May I free myself from the impact of that remark. It's not who I am."

Pause.

Stay with these loving wishes for a moment. You can also take a minute to reflect and ask if there is anything you want or need to do right now or that you might want to do later. For example, write an email to the person who hurt you or call a friend for support. Hold that with a lot of space and gentleness, too.

Pause.

Take your time with this. When you are ready, release all negative words and return to the breath for a few more minutes before you end this meditation.

14

Loving Someone with Chronic Pain*

SUFFERING FROM CHRONIC PAIN isn't hard for just the person going through it; it's also a huge challenge for anyone in a close relationship with them. If a close friend or family member has chronic pain, it will naturally have an effect on their emotional state and on your relationship. It *will* change your relationship. The closer the person is to the pain sufferer, the more strongly they will be affected. If they are both the life partner/close family member and also the caregiver, they may even be hit harder than the person in pain. Studies suggest that the partner of someone with chronic pain who is also the caregiver is even worse off than the one they are taking care of! The pain can affect all areas of their life, just as it does for the person in pain.

---

* While this book is addressed to the person suffering from pain, this chapter is aimed at their close family members or caretakers. We don't live in a vacuum, and our suffering has an effect on those who love us and help us. This chapter is for them. They are in pain because of our pain, and in return their pain is hard on us, too.

When it comes to day-to-day activities, a partner often takes over the previously shared responsibilities, like household chores and childcare. It may be that the sick partner can no longer contribute financially. This leads to a higher workload and less leisure time for the healthy partner and maybe causes them to give up on hobbies. The couple might not be able to travel as much or share other activities they previously enjoyed together. Chronic pain also tends to wreak havoc on a couple's sex life.

Because the sick partner often can't join (or predict if they will be capable of joining) a social activity, the couple will go out less often and will spend less time with friends. Over time, they'll be invited to fewer events, as others start to expect that they won't attend. Isolation (see also page 75) is real for both partners—partly because of mere exhaustion and partly because of loyalty on the part of the healthy partner.

Then there is the emotional burden. Seeing your loved one in so much pain and not being able to help causes many feelings: sadness, grief, anger, overwhelm, depression, hopelessness, and feeling stuck. These are often suppressed as the healthy partner feels that they shouldn't complain, since they're not the one with chronic pain. Caregivers who are also life partners have a higher risk of burnout than other caregivers because they're never able to take a break and get some internal (and external) distance.

Mindfulness and self-compassion can become trusted allies under these circumstances, too. Bringing kind awareness to these complex situations helps us to see more clearly what might be needed to reduce the stress and suffering of the dynamic.

Jordan and Angela have been married for thirty years and Angela has been suffering from chronic pain on and off for the last twenty years. A devoted husband and father, Jordan worked hard to make Angela's life—so radically changed by her illness—as easy as possible. When Angela started learning mindfulness, she immediately thought of Jordan. "He always feels like he needs to be the strong one and have it together all the time, but how can he? He is only human, too," she said. "But he has high blood pressure and has suffered from stomach ulcers for years. He also goes through bouts of depression. Of course, I always wondered if all of that wasn't related to his having to take care of me. I want him to learn these tools, too!"

What cares for the caregiver?

All of the ways to work with emotional pain, overwhelm, and the loss of the anticipated present and future are just the same for the loved one as for the one suffering from pain. Self-care is important—even more so for those who are caretakers. All kinds of self-care activities are helpful, especially meditation. Mindfulness (or present-moment awareness) can make other self-care activities—a workout, coffee with a friend, time out in the garden—even more effective and enhance our enjoyment of them by helping us be present and remember them clearly. The problem with self-care, though, is that it takes time. Chances are, with all the extra responsibilities that a caregiver carries, there won't be much time—or any time at all—for these wonderful activities. Massages? Nature walks? Dinner with friends? Yoga classes? Going to a game?

By all means do what you can, but know that this is not all you can do.

Here is where mindfulness and compassion come in really handy: We can practice them in any moment during our day, no matter what's going on. We don't have to say, "I'll drive you to urgent care when I come back from yoga." Mindfulness is always available, even during caretaking. You can be aware of what's going on with both your partner *and* yourself at the same time. You can see both that your partner is in pain *and* what that does to your own feelings. You can be compassionate with your partner *and* to yourself, too.

In any moment that feels right, check in with yourself: How are you feeling? How is your body feeling? Is there anything you can do right now to support yourself, like releasing the shoulders or a clenched jaw? Can you offer yourself words of kindness, like "You are doing the best you can," or acknowledge to yourself how hard this moment is: "This is a difficult moment"?

Mindfulness allows us to become aware of an emotion instead of pretending we don't have it and to acknowledge it with compassion: "A part of me feels really frustrated right now" or "There is nothing wrong with feeling the way I feel right now. This is what people feel like in this kind of situation." You are not disloyal by acknowledging how hard it is on you to be along on your loved one's pain journey. When you take care of yourself in this way, you'll notice that it becomes easier to keep showing up for your partner.

If you feel your partner's pain a lot, challenge yourself to consider the following: Is *your* pain helping your partner?

That's not to be callous—of course you will be affected by the pain your loved one is in, especially if you are a highly empathic person. But think of a person who is drowning. They don't need another person crying out in despair and jumping into the pool and drowning with them. They need someone who is compassionate and clear thinking and who will throw them a lifesaver.

Now imagine yourself in the same situation. Would you want your partner to suffer from your pain? Or would that only add to your burden? It's OK to let go of any guilt and loyalty you might be feeling. And yes, it's OK for you to feel happy and peaceful even if your partner might not! The practice in this chapter will help you gently untangle the shared pain.

What your partner needs from you, more than empathy, is *compassionate presence*.

But, you may wonder, aren't empathy and compassion the same thing? Not really, according to recent research. Empathy is an emotion that alerts you to how the other person is feeling ("I feel your pain"). You feel empathy when certain pain circuits are activated in your own brain. Compassion, on the other hand, is when you feel the pain and simultaneously experience the positive emotion of love or care, which buffers the sharp edges of the pain. Compassion becomes stronger the more we train it.

Compassion does not require the pain to disappear—although that is what we wish for—but simply arises as a natural response to pain. Compassion also carries the knowledge that there are many factors at play in someone's pain that are beyond our control. We know we can't simply make the pain go away. This understanding is further deepened in the practice of *equanimity*, or seeing the big picture, for another person (see pages 159 and 206).

This practice will help us keep the big picture in view when it comes to another person with whom we are enmeshed, whose well-being we are invested in out of love, and which causes us pain as a result. It is time that we open to the (often uncomfortable and painful) truth that we cannot make another person happy or pain free, no matter how much we want that. The words and phrases of the meditation below are helpful to use throughout your day (repeating them softly to yourself), as a reminder and "kindness anchor."

Angela eventually convinced Jordan to take a mindfulness class with her. They had a long drive to and from class, which they used to talk about what they learned. These conversations were often deep and meaningful and brought up many questions but also brought them closer together. Jordan realized how much he had been holding all those years of Angela's illness and that it was OK to take more time for himself. Angela learned to release her guilt around "ruining his life" and how to communicate her own needs for solitude and quietness more clearly.

Equanimity: every person is on their own life's journey

Start by finding a comfortable position.

Pause.

Take a moment to connect with the ground under your feet or the chair or whatever your body is resting on. Let yourself feel the support of that surface.

Pause.

If you'd like, connect with the feeling of the breath.

Pause.

How is the body feeling right now?

Pause.

Take your time to settle into this practice.

Pause.

When you're ready, bring your loved one to mind. If you'd like, picture them sitting across from you, looking at you.

Pause.

Allow yourself to feel how much you are affected by their struggle and pain.

Pause.

Now let yourself consider that every person—including your loved one and yourself—is on their own life's journey, and we cannot make another person's pain go away, despite our heartfelt wish.

Pause.

Slowly and silently repeat the following phrases to yourself:

"Everyone is on their own life's journey" or "You are on your own life's journey."

Pause.

"I am not the cause of your struggle and suffering."

Pause.

"It isn't in my power to end your suffering, although I would like to if I could."

Pause.

"Moments like this are hard to endure and yet I will continue to try to help when and where I can."

Breathe softly.

Place a hand on your chest if that comforts you.

Pause.

And repeat these phrases:

"Everyone is on their own life's journey."

Pause.

"I am not the cause of your struggle and suffering."

Pause.

"It isn't in my power to end your suffering, although I would like to if I could."

Pause.

"Moments like this are hard to endure and yet I will continue to try to help when and where I can."

Pause.

Now, when you are ready, let go of the phrases. Rest back into a bigger space of awareness, feeling the breath but with space around you, as if you could breathe beyond yourself and your loved one into the wide-open space that allows all feelings to arise and pass away.

Take a long pause.

Now come to an end of this meditation, invite movement back into the body, stretch if you like, open your eyes if you had them closed, and move on with your day.

15

Finding Your People

Shared joy is twice the joy and shared pain is half the pain.

—TRADITIONAL GERMAN PROVERB

WE ARE SOCIAL CREATURES that need to feel understood, seen, and heard. Because of this, our relationships with other people are critical to how we work mindfully with ongoing pain. Pain is a strong signal designed to occupy our full attention. Neuroscience tells us, however, that our brains have a limited attention span. So, paying "full attention" to pain can lead to not paying attention to anything else in our lives.

As a result, our relationships with the people around us—our loved ones, our family, our friends, our colleagues—can easily suffer collateral damage. When the internal noise level of the pain becomes incredibly loud, it drowns out everything else and we stop listening to others. We may start to hear and see those close to us through the lens of our own pain, which makes their actions seem careless or disrespectful of our feelings. Disconnection and loneliness deepen.

There are other factors that cause people who suffer from chronic pain to be more prone to isolation: feeling like nobody understands what you're going through; needing to spend more time with doctors and other health care providers; requiring lots of time for physical therapy simply to be able to get through the day; being tired because of the pain and the work it takes to "manage" it, which results in not having the time or energy to meet with friends or go out much at all.

Despite our pain, we're social creatures who crave and require companionship. To serve that need, we have to find ways to lessen our isolation, and a good place to start is with a little mindfulness—becoming aware of our isolation and not judging ourselves for it.

It's not your fault that your pain led to isolation, so please don't blame yourself! Offer yourself the kindness and understanding you would like from others: "It's no big surprise that I've become isolated; pain is challenging and takes up a lot of my attention."

After becoming aware of your isolation and forgiving yourself for it, you can think about what would be an easy step toward making more connection with others. A phone call? Video chat? Even just a little text message for starters? As a next step, you might also consider finding a group to support you, expanding beyond your existing network of relationships.

After years of pain and strange symptoms, Monica was diagnosed with a rare congenital connective tissue disease. While she was relieved to finally have a diagnosis and a name for her pain, it didn't make it go away. In fact, it made her feel even more strange and disconnected. She called it a freak disease. And because Monica was adopted as a baby, she had no family history to connect with. The hardest part for her was that she didn't know anybody else who suffered from this disease or had her symptoms. Her doctor suggested she find a support group.

If you suffer from a chronic condition and from chronic pain, finding others who suffer from the same ailment is helpful for most people. Support groups are often local groups that hold in-person meetings, but there are also online groups and forums where people can share and learn. It helps to be heard by people who know the details and intricacies of your condition from the inside out. It can also be gratifying to hear the experiences of others. Sometimes just being able to laugh together, or cry a little, about shared struggles can make all the difference. With today's video calling technology, online groups can be pretty effective at making the distant seem local.

In Monica's case, she checked out several online support groups and Facebook groups. She found some groups she liked, and in the midst of it all became friends with another woman with the same condition. They started to text regularly and support each other through the ups and downs of living with a chronic progressive disease. Monica had found a tribe member.

The expression "finding your tribe" suggests surrounding yourself with people who have earned your trust. They know you, love you, and understand you. When you're with them, you know you won't be judged. A tribe doesn't have to be big and the tribe members don't even have to know each other. You don't have to know every group member closely.

Your tribe doesn't have to be a formal group. It can be family members, friends, or a small community, such as your congregation or spiritual group. A public figure you follow on social media can also be part of your tribe. It might be an author or a person you admire because you really connect with what they're sharing with the world.

You do need, however, at least one or two tribe members whom you actually talk to and who know your story. The members of your tribe don't necessarily need to have the same diagnosis as you do, but it's helpful to know at least a few people who also suffer from chronic pain and who approach it in a similar way as you. There are as many different ways of coping with pain as there are forms of pain.

If mindfulness and meditation are important to you, you could try to find a mindfulness group, maybe online, for people who suffer from chronic pain. Although this is not a quick fix for your pain, finding someone who understands you and is compassionate will truly lighten your burden.

Finding strength and joy in connections with others

Start by finding a comfortable position, or as comfortable as possible. You can lie down for this meditation or sit in a chair. You can close your eyes or just soften your gaze, whatever feels best to you in this moment.

Pause.

If you are sitting, place your feet on the ground. Feel the solid ground under your feet. Sense the floor or the carpet through your shoes or bare feet.

Let your back be straight and upright, if possible, or lean back and feel the surface supporting you.

Allow the body to relax, maybe loosen the jaw, the shoulders, the belly.

Pause.

Take a few deep, slow breaths, feeling the sensations of the breath in the body, in the chest or maybe the belly.

Release a little more tension with every exhalation.

Pause.

For support, try placing a hand on your chest or on the place in the body that is hurting. Or try holding your own hand.

Pause.

Now bring to mind a friend or loved one—somebody who will bring a smile to your face by just thinking of them. Picture them in front of you, perhaps looking at you and returning your smile.

Pause.

Take a moment and think about why you love this person so much. What are their good qualities? Remember a kind or generous thing they did.

Pause.

Let yourself feel the joy and appreciation about having this person in your life.

Pause.

You can rest here, staying with this feeling. Try following this feeling even more deeply into your body to internally connect with your loved one, breathing softly.

Reflect on what you wish for this loved one. If you like, you can put those wishes into words. For example:
    May you be happy.
    May you be peaceful.
    May you be free from pain and stress and suffering.

Pause.

Now reflect for a moment about what this person wishes for *you*. Do they wish for you to be free from pain? To heal? To be healthy and strong? To be happy?

Form their wishes for you into phrases and offer them to yourself, as if you were hearing them from your friend. For example:

May you be free from pain.

May you heal.

May you be healthy and strong.

May you be happy.

Pause.

Let yourself appreciate your friend's wishes for you.

Pause.

The phrases don't have to start with "May you . . . " Perhaps "I wish for you" works better. Use whatever phrase seems natural and unforced to you. Let these wishes gently land on you like a light drizzle.

I wish for you to be free from pain.

I wish for you to heal.

I wish for you to be healthy and strong.

I wish for you to be happy

Long pause.

When you are ready, release the image of your friend, return to the breath for another minute or two, and slowly bring this meditation to an end.

PART 5

Shifting Perspective

16

The Comparing Mind

IMAGINE YOU HAVE long planned for a trip to Italy. Why Italy? Because everybody you know has either already gone or is planning to go. And it sounds wonderful! The art, the weather, the food, the culture . . . You plan and read guidebooks, buy beach clothes, and then excitedly board the plane, but when the plane lands the stewardess announces, "Welcome to Holland!" You're incredulous: What?! Holland?! This is a mistake; this can't be! You try everything to get out of there, to make it to Italy after all. But there's nothing you can do. In Holland you are and in Holland you must stay, for now. So you have to go out and buy a new guidebook and learn a whole new language (Dutch!). You get to know people you would never have met otherwise. Eventually you find that Holland is not a horrible place after all. It has tulips and even Rembrandts—it's just not what you had hoped for.

This story was first told by Emily Perl Kingsley, comforting other parents like her, with a disabled child, but the story can also be applied to chronic pain. You didn't expect to have pain that doesn't resolve. It never crossed your mind that one day you could be diagnosed with a chronic and painful disease. And yet here you are. It's natural that your mind will compare your situation with that of others.

Julia, who suffers from polyautoimmune syndrome, shares that comparing is one of the hardest pieces to deal with. "I find myself constantly comparing my situation with my friends and colleagues. I look at what they can do and where they are in their career, where they go on vacation and what they do there. And then I compare it with what I can't do and where I am in my career and life because of my illness, and that makes me feel pretty worthless and horrible."

Comparing is something that pretty much everyone does naturally. As humans we are social creatures and need to know our standing as compared to others. It's a quiet source of pain for many people who don't even carry the extra burden of chronic pain: Are we taller, shorter, or the same height? Are we more or less successful or the same? Sometimes we even do it in reverse: Who is struggling the most? Who feels the worst? "You think you have it bad? Let me tell you about *my* pain!" It's still comparing. And while it sometimes gives us a quick boost, it's doesn't last— and it leaves the other person feeling worse.

This comparing is so common, that there is a term for it in mindfulness circles: the comparing mind.

When we also suffer from chronic pain, this comparing mind easily becomes a means of self-torture. Bringing awareness to this act of comparing, we start to notice how much it hurts—and that it is actually a form of painful thinking. As we discovered in chapter 3 with the pain story, we don't have to follow the mind when it pulls in that direction. When we notice that we are comparing, we can gently note, "Ah, the comparing mind!" and come back to the breath or the feeling of the feet on the ground. We can also give ourselves compassion for pain that comparing creates in that moment: "It hurts to feel less than."

But make no mistake; the pain of the loss of the dream about Italy —the loss or the fear of the loss of your anticipated future of a healthy, pain-free body—will never fully go away. It's just too big and too significant. But if you keep comparing, keep blaming, and keep focusing on how unfair this is (it is!), then you will miss the special and beautiful things about Holland.

Releasing your comparing mind

Start by finding a comfortable position, or as comfortable as possible. You can lie down for this meditation or sit in a chair. You can close your eyes or just soften your gaze, whatever feels best to you in this moment.

Pause.

If you are sitting, place your feet on the ground. Feel the solid ground under your feet. Sense the floor or the carpet through your shoes or bare feet.

Let your back be straight and upright, if possible, or lean back and feel the surface supporting you.

Allow the body to relax, maybe loosen the jaw, the shoulders, the belly.

Pause.

Take a few deep, slow breaths, feeling the sensations of the breath in the body, in the chest or the belly.

Release a little more tension with every exhalation.

Pause.

Bring to mind a situation where you compare yourself to others in a painful way. For the purpose of this practice choose something that is mildly upsetting so that you can learn and explore the practice.

Pause.

Allow your mind to bring up the story and notice how it affects you, physically and emotionally

Pause.

Now see if you can internally step back just a little from that story and gently name or label it "Comparing Mind."

Pause.

This is the comparing mind.

Pause.

This is what the comparing mind feels like. Maybe acknowledge it with kindness:
   "It hurts to compare myself in this way!"
   "Comparing is painful!"

Use a phrase that you would offer to a hurting friend in the same situation.

Pause.

Move the attention from the pain and contraction of comparing to something more neutral, like your feet on the ground or the breath.

Pause.

Notice how the comparing mind makes you into something lesser. This is not who you are. It's like looking through distorted glasses.

There's no need to judge yourself—comparing is natural. And we can let it go.

Pause.

Repeat this process again and again if necessary. Toggle back and forth between the pain and something neutral.

Touch into the pain of comparing, noticing the painful thoughts, and then move to your breath or your feet.

Keep naming the comparing mind. Keep offering kindness.

Pause.

Now release the practice and all the comparing words and just focus on the breath for another minute or two. Bring the meditation to an end when you're ready.

17

Making Meaning

WHILE WE CAN'T CHOOSE whether or not we have pain, we can choose how we relate to it. It's up to us whether we see ourselves as a victim of unlucky circumstances or if we're open to using all of our life experiences, including pain, to grow as human beings.

As neurologist, psychiatrist, and Holocaust survivor Viktor Frankl wrote, "When we are no longer able to change a situation, we are challenged to change ourselves." Are you willing to turn the mud in your life into compost so that growth and transformation can happen? By making meaning out of your experiences, you can bear your burden with more willingness and dignity. You become an example to others, because regardless of the amount of suffering in life, we all long to live with purpose.

One way that meaning can come to us is through faith or spirituality: the belief that you have been given this challenge to learn and grow, by God, the universe, or your karma. Even if you don't believe in anything like this, you might want to consider the benefits of approaching pain as something you can learn from in order to lessen the added pain of meaninglessness.

People are naturally storytellers. Stories allow us to make sense of the world and what happens to us, and to transform that into meaning. The pain already has a story and a meaning attached to it (see page 25). We have told that story to ourselves so many times that we can't think of a different story anymore.

But it that story true?

Is it the only possible story?

Maybe you have been told a story about yourself as a child so many times that you honestly can't tell if you remember what actually happened or if you remember vivid details from the stories. A story can feel like it's true simply because we have heard it so many times. There is a classic metaphor about how the mind reacts to pain: It reacts as if we had been shot with an arrow, but instead of tending to the wound, the mind shoots a second arrow into the very same spot. If we have an injury or physical pain, instead of tending to this pain with clarity and care, the mind blasts in and multiplies the pain through judgments, resentments, resistance, and blame. You may think "I can't believe this is (still) happening! What's wrong with me? If only that driver/surgeon/fill-in-the-blanks hadn't . . ." Arrow number 1 is the pain itself. Arrow number 2 is all the thoughts and subsequent emotions that amplify the pain.

Mindfulness helps to distinguish the first and second arrows more clearly and allows us to unwedge the second arrow. This practice focuses on staying with the first arrow—the physical sensations of the pain—and not intensifying it through retelling the pain story.

Eventually we can go one step further. Since our minds are storytellers, and we need stories to make sense of our life and to move through it with purpose, we could set the intention to *shift that story* to something more meaningful. If a story can create more pain and a slew of other negative or challenging emotions, it can create the opposite, too.

Meditation teacher Thich Nhat Hanh calls this turning around of the story "No mud, no lotus." He says that just like a lotus can only grow out of the thick compost of what we call dirt or mud, in the same way the compost of broken ideas, dreams, and pain itself can tenderize and transform a heart and mind into unexpected beauty and authenticity. We don't have a choice about the loss or pain that happened to us, but we can choose how we want to learn—over time—to relate to it.

Instead of fighting the pain, we can circle back to the miracle of curiosity. When we are curious, we start paying attention again and are open to discover something new instead of clamping down on the already known. You don't need to look for an answer; instead, let an answer find you. If you are searching, you have an agenda. If you simply stroll, roam, waste time but with open ears and eyes, with an open heart, you might be surprised by something that emerges. Surprise yourself!

Vidyamala Burch, a meditation teacher, broke her back twice in her twenties, which left her with high levels of pain and a gradually increasing paralysis. During a hospital stay she came across mindfulness practice and it completely transformed her life. At the time she felt desperate, angry, helpless, and hopeless—and hated her life. Now her life is full, happy, and meaningful. No, she didn't recover from her injuries. She is confined to a wheelchair, with her lower body mostly paralyzed, including her bladder and bowel. She still has high levels of physical pain and, over time, has learned to hold all of this with kindness, equanimity, and a good sense of humor. She became a mindfulness teacher, started a training and teaching company and developed her own programs for pain, wrote a number of books, and inspired a thriving worldwide community around her. Vidyamala has now been a mindfulness practitioner for more than thirty-five years and helps others who struggle with pain. She says, "Mindfulness training has changed my life beyond all recognition and I know these simple techniques can be literally lifesaving."

Finding meaning in itself is difficult, painful, and ongoing. It can encompass many areas of your life and is not a quick fix. Growing, learning, encountering successes as well as setbacks, disappointments, and struggles is never ending.

But what are our options?

As Thich Nhat Hanh says, "The secret to happiness is to acknowledge and transform suffering, not to run away from it."

In the following meditation, I will ask you to remember a situation in your life that was very difficult at the time and that is now resolved or mostly resolved. Looking back now, you'll want to find an event that you learned from or that helped you grow.

Then we will look forward by reflecting on a current struggle. Please be kind to yourself in this practice. You can always pause and return to it later. If you'd like, have a journal ready to maybe pause the meditation throughout and jot down your thoughts. You could also journal after the meditation is over.

We call this a "silver lining reflection" from the proverb "Every dark cloud has a silver lining."

Making meaning: silver lining
backward and forward

Start by finding a comfortable position, or as comfortable as possible.

Pause.

Take a moment to connect with whatever surface your body is resting on. Let yourself feel supported.

Pause.

Connect with the feeling of the breath. The breath can be an anchor or a like a handrail to help you through challenging moments.

Pause.

How is the body is feeling right now? Maybe tired, maybe tense, maybe achy, maybe restless, maybe kind of OK, maybe all of the above or something completely different. As best as you can, allow whatever is already here to be here.

Pause.

Now I invite you to recall a situation in your life that had a silver lining; a situation that at the time was especially difficult or even unbearable. Please choose one that is now resolved or that you have come to terms with.

Think of a situation where, looking back, you understand that you learned an important lesson or felt that it tenderized you as a human being.

Pause.

Remember what happened. How did you feel about it back then? What did you believe about yourself or your life in the midst of that situation?

Pause.

And what happened instead? How did things turn out? What did it take to shift and change your feelings? What helped? What did you learn?

Pause.

Is there any advice you would give to your younger self, knowing what you know now?

Pause.

You can either pause the practice here and absorb what you've discovered or even journal about it or you may take a few deep breaths to release this situation.

Pause.

Now invite into your mind a current situation where you are struggling. View it with a sense of openness and curiosity, with gentleness and care. Step back if you notice that you can't be open or kind or if it's getting to be too much.

Pause.

Are there any similarities to how you think about the previous situation that is now resolved? This is not about the specifics of the situation, just the similarities in your thoughts and feelings.

If you find yourself thinking that it's absurd to even compare the two situations, again, please tread gently. We are looking for similar feelings about the situation, like desperation or hopelessness or a sense of failure.

Pause.

Hold these similar feelings in awareness and realize that they are a natural response to a challenging situation. It's hard to feel them. At the same time, we don't know what exactly is going to happen in the future. We know even less about how we will feel about the challenging situation as time passes.

Pause.

As lightly as you can, hold this possibility of not knowing, of letting yourself be surprised by the potential of growth and change that could be awaiting you.

Pause.

Stay here as long as you'd like if this feels good and supportive, or slowly come to the end of this reflection by releasing all of these thoughts and feelings and returning to the breath. Move on with your day.

18

The Paradox of Doing Nothing

MINDFULNESS PRACTICE TEACHES US to "be with" whatever arises in the present moment even—or especially—when that thing is challenging or painful. Learning this nonreactive, kind, and curious attention helps calm the stress reaction in the body, which in turn eases the intensity of the experience.

Doing nothing is a foreign concept to most of us. Often we feel that it's being lazy or outright bad. As a child you might have heard proverbs like "Idle hands are the devil's workshop." We are taught that if we want to learn something new, we better work hard. If we want to improve our skills, we better work hard. If something isn't the way we want it, we can work hard to change it. We put in time and effort and if that doesn't turn out the way we want it, we buckle down and try again, twice as hard. This approach is definitely helpful in many life situations.

Growing up in Germany, I learned from an early age that hard work was one of the most highly prized virtues. Sitting around and doing nothing was definitely not an option in my family. It was considered a good day when you were dog-tired in the evening from your work. My mother, who was the first female tenured professor at the college where she taught, used to say that as a woman you have to work twice as hard to achieve the same level of success as a man. Those messages go deep. At some point, they are no longer just messages. They become part of who we are.

When we are told that we should "be with" the pain, we often hear it as "doing nothing." But what is this "being with," really?

For starters, "being with" is not a passive or indifferent process. Consider taking care of a child who has the flu. We know that the flu will take as long as it takes and that we can't hurry it up by anything we do. But we will still sit with the child, maybe read them a story or sing a song, or maybe just be there for them. We know that our presence or absence at their bedside makes all the difference. Of course, we want the child to feel better and recover from the flu, but our being there is not dependent on that outcome. We are there no matter what.

Can we show up for ourselves—for the one who is in pain—in the same way? Can we keep ourselves company when we hurt and feel miserable? Loving presence is a powerful medicine whose strength we often underestimate.

Learning meditation or mindfulness does take time, discipline, and repetition, like any new skill; however, it's worth looking carefully at *the kind of effort* we are putting in. Effort in mindfulness works best when it's balanced: not too much, but not too little either.

We learn through our own direct experience how much effort is too much—where the effort tips into an attempt to force ourselves into a different experience than the one we're already having. It's natural to wish for the pain to go away and even to meditate in order for it to stop. We can apply curiosity and mindful awareness and notice: How does that feel to strive and apply force? Where does that kind of effort show up in my experience—as tension in my head, shoulders, jaw? And most of all: Is it helpful? Do I end up with the wished-for experience? Does it make the pain go away? As soon as we meditate with an agenda it will make itself known in the overall experience.

At the same time, meditating with *too little effort* is also not helpful. Here we might slip into sluggishness (which is not the same a becoming sleepy) and not care what happens with the meditation anymore, which often leads to stopping the meditation practice altogether.

In this context, then, *doing nothing* is really about inviting a sense of ease and letting insights and results come to you, rather than being lazy and avoiding what needs to be done.

Sometimes, when nothing is working, we have to take a break and rest. In sports, rest and recovery are just as essential to the performance of an athlete as training periods. During times of rest ("doing nothing"), repair, healing, rejuvenation and replenishing are happening. Because the mind and willpower are not at work, and because we can't feel the hard work that the body (and mind) is doing behind the scenes, we often dismiss the value of doing nothing and don't make enough space for it.

This resting—or doing nothing—is an essential skill that needs to be trained as much you trained its opposite (hard work) all your life.

Sometimes we need surrender. This can be a surrender to something bigger than yourself, to a higher power, to God, the universe, whatever has meaning to you. It can also be surrender to the present moment, to what is. We often associate surrender with giving up, hopelessness, a forced capitulation to what we fear or hate the most. That, of course, feels, horrible. Nobody wants to do that. Nobody wants to throw in the towel. Meditation teacher Jack Kornfield says that peace requires us to surrender our illusions of control.

Here is how I define surrender: It is the deliberate *opening, allowing, or accepting* of something that is difficult, painful, stressful, or unwanted in order to decrease the overall negative impact on ourselves and those around us. The relief of surrender is like letting yourself be joyfully carried downstream after having fought long and hard to swim upstream.

Doing nothing

Let's begin. Find a position that is as comfortable as possible.

Pause.

Can you make small adjustments to allow the body to be more relaxed?

Pause.

If you are in a seated position, feel your feet on the floor, the sup-porting ground under your feet. If you are lying down, feel any pressure of the bed or surface against your heels.

Pause.

Feel where your legs are in contact with the chair or the bed. Notice where there is touch and where there is none. Simple. Notice if your back is touching something, like the back of the chair.

Pause.

Now move your attention to the breath. Take a few long, deep breaths as if you could fill the whole body with breath.

Pause.

Inhale.

And release it.

Pause.

As always, when you notice your attention moving somewhere else, gently bring it back to wherever you are in this particular moment. Maybe silently say "Thank you, not now" to the thoughts or the distraction.

Long pause.

In your mind's eye, settle back. Imagine getting comfortable in a favorite chair. Settle in as if you were sitting outside on a lazy summer afternoon, with no to-do list and no need to be presentable for visitors.

Feel the space in front of and around you and open that spaciousness in your inner experience.

Pause.

If you experience pain in this moment, observe it as just one part of the bigger picture. You don't need to do anything right now. Allow yourself to not fix it or change it.

Pause.

Remember a time of leisure that felt pleasant and easy. What made it so?

Pause.

Allow yourself to feel into what pleasant and easy *would* feel like.

Take this moment to slow down, to unwind any sense of busyness or pressure you might feel right now.

You might find it helpful to slow down the breath. Invite your whole body, your whole system, to gradually slow down and relax.

Pause.

If thoughts arise that tell you not to relax, allow them to move into the background. Don't engage with them. Come back to the sense of slowing down and opening up, of relaxing.

Remember that you have already set aside this time to meditate. Can you meditate as a way for your whole being to pause and rest—and to actually do nothing?

Can you allow yourself to take in this time of respite, of ease, despite everything that's going on in your body and in your life?

Pause.

If you feel resistance, notice where there is tension in the body. Try to soften that feeling a little, like muscles soften when submerged in warm water.

Pause.

Imagine breathing into areas of tightness or discomfort, which can also help to soften, to unwind.

Pause.

Notice where there might be tension in your mind, maybe felt as tension in your head or your jaw. Can you soften your mind?

Pause.

Ease the burden of the stories you might be carrying and breathe deeply. Nothing needs to be done right now; there's nothing to accomplish.

Pause.

Being here and feeling whatever you are feeling right now is enough.

Pause.

Do you need to work hard to feel?

Just like we don't need to work hard to see or to hear, feeling comes naturally. You can just lean back and let it come.

Allow whatever is arising to move through you, like a river or the wind moves through a landscape.

Long pause.

When you are ready, slowly let this meditation end. Invite movement back into the body, maybe stretching, if that feels right. And move on with your day.

19

The Big Picture

PAIN IS the body's way of telling the brain, "Pay attention!" Since it secures the body's safety, pain will always take top priority when it comes to the brain's attention. That makes sense with acute pain, since it's telling the brain to be careful, so you don't do further damage, and to be aware of the area that needs healing. When it comes to chronic pain, however, that high-priority status doesn't work in our favor: The alarm is sounding but there's nothing to be done. On top of that, we don't seem to build up much tolerance to pain over time. We get used to other stimuli, like sounds or sights, but we don't get used to pain. Pain just keeps hurting.

Having chronic pain is like being in a beautiful garden, but only able to see the one plant that is sickly and not thriving, which causes us to forget about the rest. Even if most of our body is fine, if we have chronic pain, then it commands our attention and can blot out everything else.

Mindfulness practice is useful because it trains and directs our attention, allowing us the choice about what we spotlight. Mindfulness has the capacity to *zoom in*, to examine the details of an experience, or to *zoom out* and see the whole picture. Left to its own devices, our nervous system will automatically zoom in on the pain, which will make it seem like there is nothing else going on in our body besides it. Let's say your shoulder is hurting. Doesn't that make you feel like feel like all you are is that painful shoulder?

Brian came to me because of exactly that: a frozen shoulder that wouldn't resolve. This condition and its treatment kept Brian constantly focused on his left shoulder. He worried a lot about the pain and anticipated how each day would go based on expected bouts of pain.

Mindfulness training teaches us how to open the lens of awareness so that we become unstuck from the limited world of pain. We check for sensations—pain or no pain—starting with just one other part of the body and eventually including the entire body. How much of your body is actually in pain: 5 percent? 10 percent? 30 percent? In that case then, 95 percent, 90 percent, or 70 percent of the body is pain free! Rarely is the entire body in pain.

Brian and I did body scans together in which he learned to expand his focus to all areas of his body, not just the shoulder. Whenever his attention would go to the shoulder, he would acknowledge it and then refocus on wherever he was in the body scan. Except for his shoulder, the rest of his body was usually completely pain free. That realization offers huge relief—to not only *know* that most of your body is pain free but to also *feel* it.

Once we have explored the entire body in this way, we can zoom out beyond physical boundaries of the body to include a bigger perspective: We can become aware of the space around us, the room we are in, the house. This can be done either with the eyes closed, feeling the space around you, or with eyes open, taking in the space around you, deliberately and slowly.

Brian liked to do this practice at home in his backyard, sitting on a favorite chair. He said, "I like to first sit with my eyes open, taking in the trees and shrubs and flowers. Then when I close my eyes I can kind of still feel this aliveness of my garden around me. This somehow lets the shoulder pain just be there as a part of me and my whole garden. Those are very peaceful moments!"

You can draw on the space around you to invite in awareness of other areas in your life that are beautiful and thriving. What can you include here? Family? Friends? Things you enjoy or love to do despite the pain? What are you passionate about?

When Brian reflected on his life, he realized that he had a lot of healthy, beautiful plants not simply in his actual garden but also in the garden of his life: His partner, their kids and grandkids, their dog, good friends, his passion for watching hockey games.

If you take a spoonful of salt and put it in a glass of water, the water will taste very salty, but if you take that same spoonful of salt and put it in a lake, you won't be able to taste the salt at all. This is a classic analogy in meditation. Just as it's not about the amount of salt but the size of the container, try to experience your pain in the biggest possible container. In this way we can move from focusing on the one sickly plant in the garden of our life and instead take in the garden in its entirety and rest in the overall beauty.

The big picture

Find a comfortable position. Feel the connection the body has with the ground.

Is there any tension you can let go of to allow all other sensations to be present?

Pause.

Connect with the breath and take a few deep, slow breaths.

Pause.

Now place the attention on an area that is in pain or discomfort right now. Feel what is here without overwhelming yourself.

If you find it helpful for support, place a hand on your chest or on the part that is in pain to convey that you are not just paying attention but rather kind attention.

Pause.

Now can you imagine using the breath to either breathe into the pain and soften it or to breathe around it?

Pause.

Take your time.

Pause.

When you are ready, let the lens of your awareness expand to include the areas around the pain.

Widen the lens of awareness to reach more and more areas of the body without letting go of the painful part. See if they are in pain. Hold the painful and not-painful parts at the same time.

Pause.

You can always return to the breath or pause for a moment if you need to, and open your eyes, look around, then continue when you feel ready.

Pause.

Feel into the body until you have a sense of the entire body—but without focusing on specific details. See the forest for the trees.

Pause.

Allow everything to be the way it is in this moment.

Pause.

Stay with this exploration as long as you'd like. You might need to readjust from time to time if the mind gets stuck in details again.

Pause.

Try to expand beyond your body and include people and areas of support in your expansive view: family, friends, your care team, things you enjoy or are passionate about.

Feel into this big picture of your life, in all its imperfection and complexity.

Pause.

Stay with this for a few minutes before you release the big picture and come back to just feeling the breath and the body again.

Pause.

Take your time to transition, opening your eyes and closing the meditation when you are ready.

20

Stop Trying to Get Better

Don't aim at success. The more you aim at it and make it a target,
the more you are going to miss it. For success,
like happiness, cannot be pursued. . . . Happiness must happen, and
the same holds for success: You have to let it
happen by not caring about it.

—VIKTOR FRANKL, *MAN'S SEARCH FOR MEANING*

ELIMINATING TRYING might be the most controversial of all reflections and practices shared here, so at the outset, I ask you to try to stay as open-minded as possible while reading through this chapter, giving it some thought and time to sink in.

Many people come to meditation because they want to learn how to relax. So what do they do when they find themselves meditating and can't relax? They are frustrated—and then try harder! As it turns out, the result of trying hard to relax—whether through meditation or otherwise—is not relaxation. The goal of mindfulness is not to relax—the goal is to be present with whatever is arising, moment by moment. It's OK to not be relaxed.

Quite often just that little bit of permission makes it possible to relax. It's similar with falling asleep: What happens when you try to force yourself to fall asleep? *Not* falling asleep! We have to set the conditions for falling asleep—and then we need to let go.

That's exactly the twist I invite you to consider here. Psychologist Carl Rogers said, "The curious paradox is that when I accept myself just as I am, then I can change." The struggle to *get better*—while completely normal and understandable—often gets in the way of our feeling OK right now. It suggests that as long as we are not pain free we cannot be OK. This places a big constraint on everything we experience and ends up holding us back. It also keeps our system held in a constant state of rejection, struggle, and stress.

Research shows that the more relaxed and stress free we are, the faster we can heal. Stress suppresses the immune system; when we are stressed our ability to heal slows down. Here comes our paradox:

> *Can we allow ourselves to stop working so desperately on healing in order to promote healing?*

> *If healing might not be possible, can we still learn to be OK wherever we are?*

Time and again people have told me that stress worsens their condition or accelerates flare-ups. And suffering from chronic pain is stressful on many levels: managing symptoms, going to multiple doctors or therapist appointments, extra time and costs, strain on social life . . . the list goes on. Yet the overarching stressor may well be the fear that our condition will not get better and might even get worse. Facing this reality, we tend to jump to the conclusion that we will never be happy again, never feel OK again. On top of that, our mind conjures up worst-case scenarios to counteract the uncertainty. And because our body doesn't differentiate between real and imagined fear, the stress response in the body is the same.

What if you could find a way to let that stress go?

What if you only had to deal with the real problems at hand, and not with the anticipated ones?

Bonnie, who suffers from interstitial cystitis said to me, "It's not that I don't care about the pain anymore. I still do, of course, and pain has a way of grabbing your attention, no matter what. But I realized that if I put the rest of my life and my happiness on hold until the pain is gone, I might end up empty-handed. There is a real possibility that my condition will never completely resolve. It does in some people and it doesn't in others. So I really feel I have to take my happiness and dreams into my own hands. It's up to me."

I'm not asking you to stop caring whether you get healthy; not at all. But I invite you to imagine what could change if you weren't so hyper-focused on a specific outcome.

This brings us to the interesting question of what we actually mean by *healing*? Is it the same as being cured? The philosopher S. Kay Toombs, who herself suffered from multiple sclerosis, asks us to consider healing as a *restoration of wholeness*, which *may* include the curing of the disease but is *not limited to it*. Wholeness relates to the ability to preserve one's integrity in the face of the pain or the disease. We can choose to live well in the presence of our condition, rather than being defined by its absence.

Zen teacher Ezra Bayda expresses a similar idea when he says, "We often think that being healed means the illness and the pain will go away. But healing doesn't necessarily mean that the physical body will mend. . . . Healing is not just about physical symptoms. Many people heal and still remain physically sick or even die. Many who become physically well never really heal. Healing involves clearing the pathway to the open heart. . . . To heal, to become whole, we no longer identify with ourselves as just this body, as just our suffering. We identify with a vaster sense of being." That *sense of being* that we all possess is focused not on a future condition that we long to have but on our present reality.

My wish for you is that—regardless of whether or not you have pain—you can live your life to the fullest right here, right now. There's no need to stop planning to take care of your future, but may you do so with openness and ease, staying mostly *here*, in the present moment, and making the best of it.

OK as you are

Start by finding a comfortable position, or as comfortable as possible.

Pause.

Take a moment to connect with the ground beneath you. Let yourself feel the support of that surface.

Pause.

If you like, connect with the feeling of the breath.

Pause.

How is the body feeling right now?

Pause.

Notice how you feel about how you're feeling right now. If you are OK, become aware of that feeling and rest with it. Try breathing with the sense of being OK.

Pause.

If you are not feeling OK, can you seek out where that feeling lives? Become curious. Where do you not feel OK?

Is it in a particular location in the body? In one area or in several?

How would you describe that feeling? Is it a form of tension? Does it have a texture? Do you know where it originates?

Pause.

Notice if there is also a layer of resistance. If so, is that a resistance to not being OK, or is it the resistance itself that is at the core of not feeling OK?

Come back to the breath to slow down. Investigate with curiosity as well as kindness.

Pause.

Now see if you can locate the wish to get better, to heal. How does that wish show up in your experience? Is it in your head? Can you locate it somewhere in your body? Is it a feeling of pressure or urgency? Or is it a sense of ease and deep caring? Maybe it's something else completely. Where do you feel it? In the area of your heart? Somewhere else?

Pause.

If there is a sense of pressure or urgency, what would happen if—just for now—you let that go? Let go of the need to be any different from how you already are. How does that feel? What would change?

Pause.

Invite the possibility to be OK as you are. Right in this moment.

Pause.

This might feel foreign, but that doesn't mean it's wrong or that you can't learn it.

Pause.

Let go of all thoughts and contemplations. Simply rest back into a bigger space beyond all sensations, feelings, and thoughts. Feel the rhythm of the breath or focus on nothing in particular other than this spacious place.

Pause.

In your own time, let this meditation end and move on with your day.

EPILOGUE

Closing Thoughts

I TRULY HOPE that this little book has brought some new insights and more ease into your life. We have revealed glimpses into quite complex topics. Sometimes a glimpse is enough to spark a transformation; sometimes we need to spend more time with the idea and the practices.

To move forward, use what you find helpful and consider returning to topics that might have felt foreign or even counterintuitive on the first read. You might feel complete with reading these chapters and doing the meditations and reflections, or you might feel inspired to learn more about a particular topic through books or by taking a mindfulness class. Most people benefit from some form of regular meditation practice, time dedicated to just being present without the added bustle of everyday life, our phones, people, or our never-ending to-do lists. Establishing a daily meditation like Mindfulness of the Breath or Mindfulness of Sound is a great foundation for then revisiting any of the practices in this book as needed.

Relating to pain through the lens of kind awareness opens space and releases stories and emotions that are not serving us anymore.

Sometimes transformation comes quickly, and sometimes it takes its sweet time. I remember the relief I felt when I first understood that my thoughts don't define who I am! Of course I still often forget this and need a reminder. But that is simply part of my ongoing practice. I know this kind of freedom is possible and available to all of us.

I wish from my heart that your pain will resolve and heal as fast as possible! May this book become a trusted companion on your path toward wholeness and integration. May this book become something that you have marked with sticky notes and penciled observations and that you keep close by as you travel on your journey. May what you learn spill over to touch your entire life, not just your relationship with your physical pain.

Many people who first came to me because of their pain have reported that their relationships with their partners, kids, or coworkers have changed for the better through these practices. Mindfulness and compassion are true allies. What we start out as doing for ourselves we end up doing for all of us. And that's what the world needs more of: for us to be awake and alive with meaning and joy.

Audio recordings of the guided meditations in this book can be found at christianewolf.com/oyp/audio.

You can also access the audio files by scanning this QR code with the camera on your phone or a QR reader app.

RESOURCES

RESOURCES ON PAIN

Bernhard, Toni. *How to Live Well with Chronic Pain and Illness: A Mindful Guide*. Somerville, MA: Wisdom Publications, 2015.

Burch, Vidyamala, and Danny Penman. *You are Not your Pain: Using Mindfulness to Relieve Pain, Reduce Stress, and Restore Well-Being*. New York: Flatiron Books, 2015.

RESOURCES ON MINDFULNESS

Collard, Patrizia. *The Little Book of Mindfulness: 10 Minutes a Day to Less Stress, More Peace*. London: Gaia, 2014.

Greater Good magazine, greatergood.berkeley.edu.

Kabat-Zinn, Jon. *Wherever You Go, There You Are: Mindfulness Meditation in Everyday Life*. New York: Hachette Books, 2005.

Kornfield, Jack. *No Time Like the Present: Finding Freedom, Love, and Joy Right Where You Are*. New York: Atria Books, 2018.

mindful: mindful.org

RESOURCES ON SELF-COMPASSION

Brach, Tara. *Radical Compassion: Learning to Love Yourself and Your World with the Practice of RAIN.* New York: Viking, 2019.

Neff, Kristin, and Christopher Germer. *The Mindful Self-Compassion Workbook: A Proven Way to Accept Yourself, Build Inner Strength, and Thrive.* New York: Guilford Press, 2018.

Neff, Kristin. *Self-Compassion: The Proven Power of Being Kind to Yourself.* New York: HarperCollins, 2011.

MINDFULNESS MEDITATION APPS

Insight Timer: guided meditations, programs, or just a timer with a bell

Headspace: guided meditations, programs

Calm: guided meditations, programs

10% Happier: guided meditations, programs, and podcast

ACKNOWLEDGMENTS

With much appreciation and affection for the following:

All the people who have taken classes with me over the years, who came with their physical or emotional pain and whose sharing and stories profoundly influenced my own learning and fine-tuning of these teachings. I am particularly grateful to Denise Bardovi, who has honored me with sharing her ongoing pain journey over many years, which, in return, helped me to midwife many new insights around this tender and tough topic.

Batya Rosenblum, senior editor at The Experiment, who immediately grasped my idea and intention with this book and helped every step of the way to bring it to life. I'm particularly grateful to her skillful and thoughtful editing.

Juliann Barbato and Zach Pace for their copyediting magic.

Stephany Evans, my agent, whose clear guidance helped me find the perfect fit for the book.

Barry Boyce, friend, colleague, fellow practitioner, and developmental editor for his clear and precise feedback and fine-tuning. He shared many insights about book writing and editing and we enjoyed many dharma-mindfulness discussions.

Dan Siegel, fellow MD turned awareness teacher, author, and pack leader, for his support and wonderful foreword.

Charles "Chuck" Mondry for coming up with the awesome title. None of the other options came even close!

Greg Serpa, my dear friend and longtime partner in crime for teaching and developing new programs at the VA (US Department of Veterans Affairs)—our brains combined are simply better than individually!

Trudy Goodman and Jack Kornfield for their "spiritual parenting." Trudy, I'm so grateful for your continued friendship, support, and mentorship! And for our walks and ocean swims.

My wonderful InsightLA family of fellow teachers, our awesome office team, and our community of fellow practitioners. And my loving circle of friends and my sister Iris: Thank you for letting me be myself!

My biggest thank you goes to my husband, Bert, for his unwavering loving support, and to our kids, Lynn, Tristan, and Antonia.

And last but not least to my running community, whose commitment and positivity help me stay sane (and in training) during the craziness of 2020.

Meditation Acknowledgments

Self-compassion meditation, on page 54, is adapted from a meditation in the Mindful Self-Compassion (MSC) curriculum.

Urge surfing meditation, on page 116, is adapted from a meditation in the Mindfulness-Based Relapse Prevention (MBRP) curriculum.

Forgiveness meditation, on page 136, is adapted from a meditation by Jack Kornfield.

Equanimity meditation, on page 159, is adapted from a meditation in the Mindful Self-Compassion (MSC) curriculum.

ABOUT THE AUTHOR

CHRISTIANE WOLF, MD, PHD is a physician turned mindfulness and compassion teacher and a senior teacher at InsightLA (InsightLA.org) in Los Angeles, California. She trains teachers and teaches Mindfulness-Based Stress Reduction (MBSR) and Mindful Self-Compassion to groups and individuals in the US and across Europe. With her medical background, one of her specialties is working with people who suffer from chronic illness and pain. Dr. Wolf is a lead teacher and program developer for the nationwide mindfulness facilitator training for the US Veterans Administration.

Dr. Wolf is also a Buddhist teacher in the Vipassana (Insight) meditation tradition and has received teacher transmission from Trudy Goodman and Jack Kornfield. She is the coauthor, with Greg Serpa, of *A Clinician's Guide to Teaching Mindfulness*. Dr. Wolf lives in Los Angeles with her husband and their three children.

christianewolf.com | ⊙christianewolfmindfulness